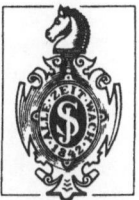

Thian Lok Tio

Endosonography in Gastroenterology

With 115 Figures and 26 Tables

Springer-Verlag
Berlin Heidelberg New York
London Paris Tokyo

T. Lok Tio
Acad. Med. Centre
University of Amsterdam
Div. of Gastroenterology – Hepatology
Meibergdreef 9
NL-1105 AZ Amsterdam

ISBN-13: 978-3-540-19434-7   e-ISBN-13: 978-3-642-73837-1
DOI: 10.1007/978-3-642-73837-1

For Ting Soan
Hong-Xia
Xiao-Rui

Contents

Introduction

Transcutaneous ultrasonography is an established procedure for diagnosis and therapy in gastroenterology. However, ultrasonic images can often be hampered by pulmonary and intestinal gas and by bony and adipose tissue. In 1956 Wild and Reid reported the first results of transrectal ultrasound of the prostate [1]. In 1976 Lutz introduced an A-mode ultrasonic probe which could be introduced via the biopsy channel of an endoscope [2]. In 1978 and 1980 Hisanaga performed echocardiography using an ultrasonic transducer attached to the tip of a flexible instrument [3, 4]. In animal studies and later on in humans Di Magno has used an echoendoscope in which a small transducer was attached at the tip of a fiberoptic endoscope [5, 6]. The purpose was to overcome the limitations of transcutaneous ultrasonography by directly approaching target lesions with a high-frequency ultrasound source via the gastrointestinal lumen. Subsequently, the first series of endoscopic ultrasonography (EUS) examinations were reported during the European congress in Stockholm [7]. The purpose of this book is:

1. To evaluate the technique and the equipment for endoscopic ultrasonography
2. To evaluate in detail the endosonographic pattern of the normal and abnormal wall structure
3. To analyze a large consecutive series of various gastrointestinal malignancies in order to determine the usefulness and accuracy of EUS in the detection, staging, and therapy of malignant diseases
4. To compare EUS with other imaging techniques

References

1. Wild JJ, Reid JM (1956) Br J Phys Med 19: 248–257
2. Lutz H, Roesch W (1976) Transgastroscopic Ultrasonography. Endoscopy 8: 203–205
3. Hisanaga K, Hisanaga A (1978) A new real-time sector scanning system of ultra-wide angle and real-time recording of entire cardiac images: transesophagus and transchest methods. Ultrasound Med 4: 391–402
4. Hisanaga K, Hisanaga A, Hibi N et al. (1980) High speed rotating scanner for transesophageal cross-sectional echocardiography. Am J Cardiol 46: 837
5. Di Magno EP, Buxton JL, Regan PT et al. (1980) The ultrasonic endoscope. Lancet: 629–31
6. Di Magno EP, Silverstein F, Giuliani D, Ohnmori S (1982) An improved ultrasonic endoscope: preliminary canine experiments (abstr.). Gastrointest Endosc 28: 129–130
7. Classen M, Kawai K (1984) Scand J Gastroenterol; 19 (suppl 102): 5–37
8. Classen M, Kawai K (1984) Scand J Gastroenterol; 19 (suppl 94): 1–10
9. Tytgat GNJ, Tio TL (1986) Scand J Gastroenterol; 21 (suppl 123): 1–169
10. Heyder N, Lutz H, Lux G (1983) Ultraschalldiagnostik via Gastroskop. Ultraschall Med 4: 84–93

11. Lux G, Heyder N, Demling L (1982) Endoscopic Ultrasonography
12. Di Magno EP, Regan PT, Clain JE, James EM, Buxton JL (1982) Human endoscopic ultrasonography. Gastroenterology 83: 824–829
13. Lux G, Heyder N, Demling L (1982) Endoscopic ultrasonography – technique, orientation and diagnostic possibilities. Endoscopy 4: 220–225
14. Heyder N, Lutz H, Lux G (1983) Ultraschalldiagnostik via Gastroskop. Ultraschall Med 4: 84–93
15. Strohm WD, Classen M (1984) Endosonographie mit einem Gastrofiberskop. Ultraschall Med 5: 84–93
16. Tio TL, Tytgat GNJ (1984) Endoscopic ultrasonography in the assessment of intra- en transmural infiltration of tumours in the oesophagus, stomach and papilla of Vater and in the detection of extraoesophageal lesions. Endoscopy 4: 220–225
17. Caletti G, Bolondi L, Brocchi P et al. (1983) Staging of gastric cancer by means of endoscopic ultrasonography (abstr). Gastroenterology 84: 13866
18. Tio TL, den Hartog Jager FCA, Tytgat GNJ (1986) Endoscopic ultrasonography of Non-Hodgkin lymphoma of the stomach. Gastroenterology 91: 401–408
19. Tio TL, Tytgat GNJ (1986) Atlas of transintestinal ultrasonography. Mur Kostverloren BV, Aalsmeer, The Netherlands

I Instruments and Technique of Investigation

Since 1983 we have been using an Olympus prototype echoendoscope (EU-M1) and in later stages the commercially available echoendoscope (EU-M2). The length of the rigid tip is 45 mm (EU-M1) or 42 mm (EU-M2). The frequency of the real-time ultrasonic beam is 7.5 MHz and it has a penetration depth of approximately 10 cm and a theoretical axial resolution of 0.2 mm.

Recently we started to use an Olympus prototype instrument with a frequency of 10 MHz. The penetration depth of the ultrasound in the latter instrument is approximately 5 cm and it has a theoretical axial resolution of 0.1 mm. The motor of the mechanical scanner is attached to the proximal part of the endoscope. The transducer attached to the tip of side-viewing endoscope is routinely covered with a water-filled balloon to improve the ultrasonic image by making optimal contact with the mucosa. In case of extensive stenosis which cannot be passed with the echoendoscope (outer diameter 13 mm) a flexible nonfiberoptic Aloka prototype instrument is available with a diameter of 10 mm and a frequency of 7.5 MHz. This instrument is technically compatible with the Olympus echoendoscope. However, there is no possibility for optical viewing or for maneuvering the transducer upward or downward from the axis. By rotating the instrument the transducer can be moved around its axis.

For transrectal investigation two instruments are available:
1. An instrument with a rigid shaft, 12 cm long, with a transducer attached at the tip. The diameter of the transducer is 15 mm. The instrument is routinely covered with a water-filled balloon.
2. A flexible Aloka prototype instrument, which has been described above.

For transsigmoidal investigation we have used the Olympus echoendoscope in order to pass the rectosigmoid junction and to introduce the instrument as deeply as possible.

Technique of Investigation

The Upper Gastrointestinal (GI) tract

After anesthetizing the throat and sedating with diazepam (7.5–10 mg), the echoendoscope is inserted like any other endoscope with the patient in the left lateral position. The echoendoscope is blindly introduced in the esophagus and then further down into the stomach.

Esophagus

For investigation of the esophagus only the water-filled balloon method can be used. Using information usually gathered after prior routine endoscopy, the echoprobe can be placed in the area of the lesion by measuring the distance between the tip of the instrument and the teeth. After adequate filling of the balloon with deaerated (boiled) water, the lesion can be placed into the focus of the ultrasonic beam to achieve clear ultrasonic images. Not only the primary lesion but also adjacent structures such as lymph nodes, vascular structures, and adjacent organs should be carefully identified. In case of esophageal cancer the instrument should be introduced into the stomach in order to visualize lymph nodes at the celiac axis, along the lesser curvature of the stomach, and in the splenic hilum and cardia. During withdrawal of the instrument, particularly in the cervical part of the esophagus, the water should be removed from the balloon in order not to compress the trachea and to avoid patients' feeling any discomfort. In case of extensive stenosis the flexible Aloka instrument can be introduced into the narrowed area. Using ultrasonic images the instrument should be gently introduced as deeply as possible.

Stomach

In the investigation of the stomach accurate placing of the transducer on the lesion is mandatory to obtain adequate ultrasonic images. Because the direction of ultrasound is perpendicular to the axis of the instrument and identical with the optical direction of side-viewing optics the target lesion should first be found endoscopically to place the echoprobe accurately on the target and then sonographically. Mucous and bilious staining must be removed endoscopically to achive a clear ultrasonic image. Thereafter the space between the transducer and the mucosa should be filled with water to produce adequate transmission of ultrasound. Two methods are available:
1. A water-filled balloon method, in which deaerated water is instilled into a balloon attached to the tip of the instrument.
2. A water-filled stomach method, in which water is introduced into the gastric lumen via the biopsy channel of the echoendoscope. For lesions in the corpus and fundus of the stomach we prefer the water-filled stomach method because a clear image can be obtained of the intraluminal and longitudinal extent of any abnormality. Lesions in the antrum and cardia of the stomach which cannot adequately be coated with water should be examined by filling the balloon and the GI lumen with water.

For standardizing transverse ultrasonic images, the pancreas should be placed at the bottom, the liver on the right side, and the spleen on the left side of the screen, similar to the conventional position for computed tomography (CT). Longitudinal sections should be made by placing the liver on the right side and the pancreas and spleen on the left side of the screen. In general, the cranial part of the body should be positioned towards the upper side and the caudal part towards the lower side of the screen. Before removal of the instrument the water should be removed from the stomach to avoid aspiration.

Duodenum

After visualizing the pylorus the instrument is gently inserted into the duodenal bulb in a way similar to the technique usually used in endoscopic retrograde cholangiopancreatography (ERCP). However, maneuvering into the duodenum is usually more difficult when compared to ERCP due to the lenght of the rigid tip. The ultrasonic unit should not be switched on whilst maneuvering the instrument into the duodenum. Occasionally, insertion into the second part of the duodenum can be extremely difficult or even impossible, particularly in the presence of duodenal deformity due to ulcer disease, pancreatitis, or pancreatic cancer. After passing the duodenal bulb the instrument should be introduced as far as possible. The transducer should be placed adequately on the lesion under endoscopic monitoring. The water-filled balloon method is to be preferred because the instilled water rapidly disappears into the distal part of the duodenum. In case of extensive polypoid or exophytic lesions, however, rapidly filling the lumen with water may allow clear visualization of the intraluminal extent of the lesions. For standardizing ultrasonic images the caval vein, vertebra, and aorta should be placed in the lower part and the liver on the right side of the screen, in a way similar to that used for CT.

Pancreas

Because of the anatomical topographic relationship between the pancreas, stomach, and duodenum, a transgastric and transduodenal approach should provide accurate visualization of the entire pancreas. For the transgastric approach the configuration of the stomach is important. An elongated stomach allows excellent visualization of the entire pancreas. In contrast, a small, contracted stomach or a partially resected stomach makes adequate examination of the pancreas difficult or even impossible because the head of the pancreas cannot be reached with the transducer and because of the limited penetration depth of high-frequency ultrasound. Usually the head and particularly the periampularry region must be examined from the second part of the duodenum. The body and the tail of the pancreas have to be examined from the middle and proximal part of the stomach. The most important landmark in the transgastric approach is the splenic vein, which can be found by placing the transducer along the posterior wall of the middle part of the stomach. Teh pancreatic parenchyma is visualized as a finely granular echopattern immediately above the splenic vein.

For the transduodenal approach the caval vein, vertebra, and aorta are the most important landmarks. Using these landmarks for orientation the instrument can slowly be withdrawn until the entire head of the pancreas is visualized. The uncinate process can usually be identified as a hooked echopattern continuous with parenchyma of the head of pancreas adjacent to the caval vein and mesenteric vessels. The distal part of the portal vein, the splenoportal junction, and the superior mesenteric vein are also important for orientation and particularly for staging of malignant disease. The periampullary region can be identified as a polypoid structure and the pancreatic duct and/or the bile duct are immediately adjacent to the duodenal lumen.

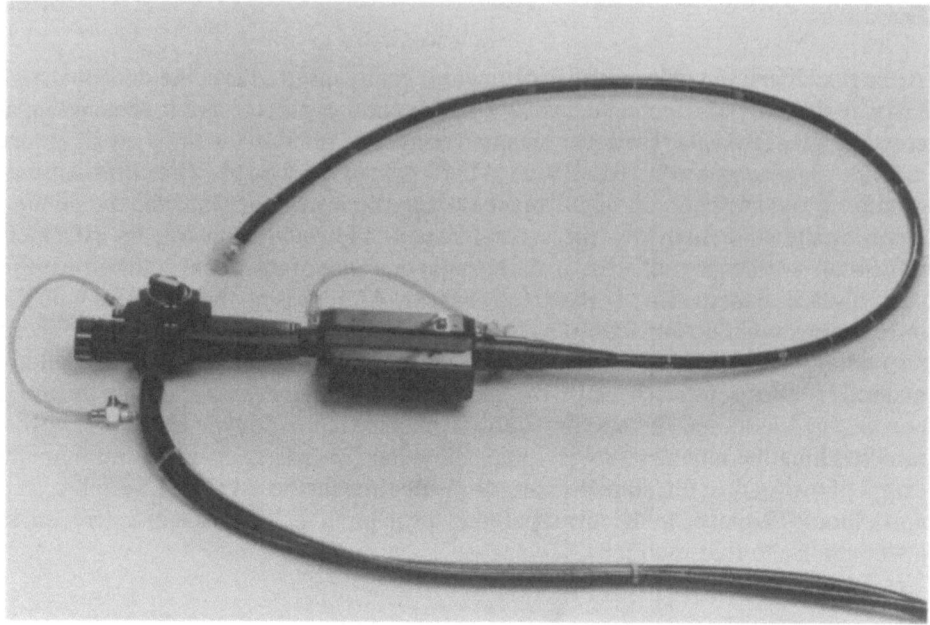

Fig. 1. Echoendoscope (Olympus EUM2) consisting of a side viewing gastroscope JFB3 with a small echoprobe (e) at its tip and a motor (m) of the rotatig sector system of ultrasound channel for filling the gastric (g) lumen on the balloon (b) with water

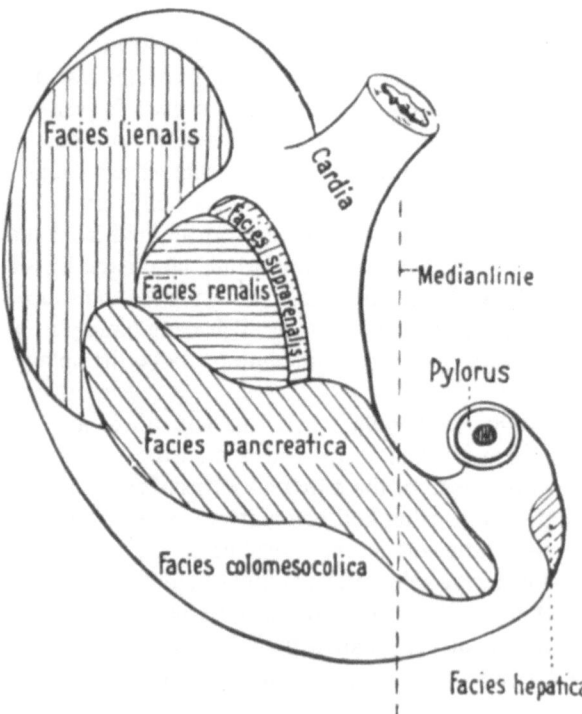

Fig. 3. Anatomic scheme (posterior view) shows the relationship between the stomach and the surrounding organs. Note the localisation of the pancreas at the posterior wall of antrum and corpus of the stomach

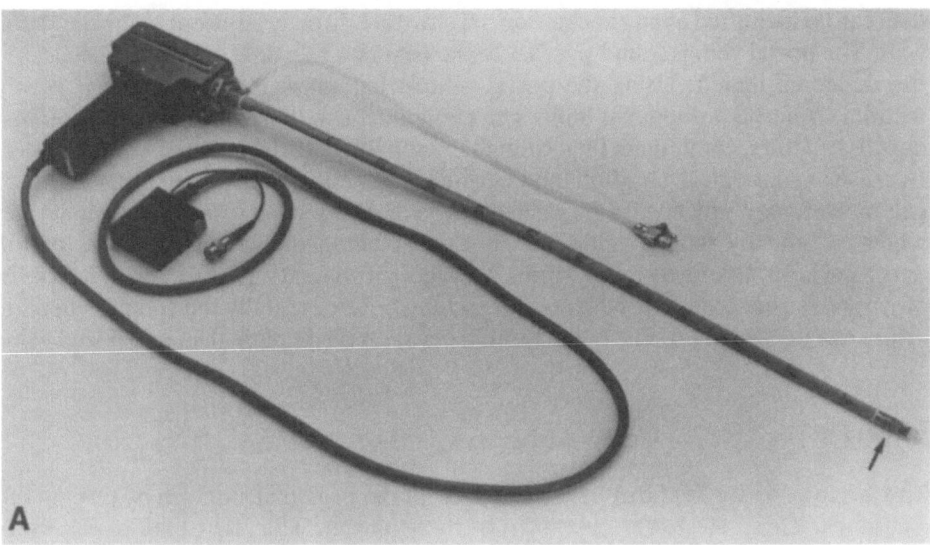

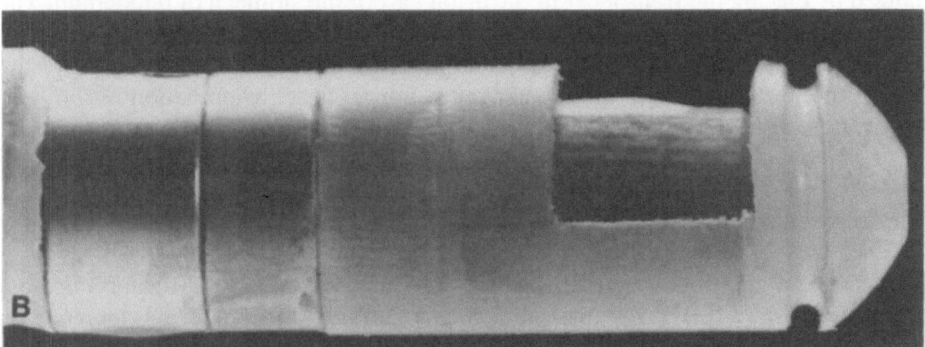

Fig. 2. A Flexible non-optic ALOKA instrument with a small echoprobe at its tip; B Magnification view of the echoprobe

The pancreatic duct (Wirsung's duct) can be visualized starting from the periampullary region up to the tail of the pancreas. Occasionally Santorini's duct can be identified approximately 1 cm above and ventrally from the periampullary region. In the body and tail of the pancreas the pancreatic duct is seen as an anechoic structure with a hyperechoic echopattern from the adjacent parenchyma, that is almost parallel to the splenic vein at a distance of nearly 1 cm and that is always oriented in a ventral direction.

The Biliary System

For investigation of the distal biliary system including the periampullary region the trancducer must be inserted into the second part of the duodenum. The common bile duct can be identified as an anechoic ductal structure directly adjacent to the duodenal wall. The portal vein is found parallel to the common bile duct and more distal from the duodenal lumen. Using the portal vein as landmark the instrument is slowly withdrawn into the duodenal bulb. The cystic duct can be seen as a serpentine-like ductal structure communicating with the common bile duct and the gallbladder. Because of anatomical variations and the limited penetration depth of ultrasound, the gallbladder may not always be visualized using the portal vein as an orientation landmark and by maneuvering the transducer along the lesser curvature of the duodenal bulb and the distal stomach. Adjacent intrahepatic portal veins can be seen directly adjacent to and distal from the GI lumen. Occasionally the common hepatic artery can be identified, this being located between hepatic duct and portal vein.

Liver

The left lobe of the liver can be examined from the proximal stomach by placing the transducer along the lesser curvature of the stomach. The right lobe of the liver, particularly the quadrate lobe and the area adjacent to the GI lumen, can be visualized by placing the transducer in the distal part of the stomach or duodenum. The entire right lobe of the liver, however, cannot be seen because of the limited penetration depth of the ultrasound. The most important landmark for examination of the liver is the portal vein and the hepatic veins. For accurate examination of the liver transcutaneous ultrasound is mandatory.

The Rectum and Rectosigmoid Region

For rectal examination we prefer to use a rigid instrument with 5 MHz or a flexible echoprobe with 7.5 MHz. After cleaning the rectum with phosphate or a water enema the instrument in gently inserted as deep as possible in a way similar to that used in sigmoidoscopy. After filling the balloon with water the instrument can slowly be withdrawn using the ultrasonic image as orientation. For standardizing ultrasound images the prostate gland or the uterus must be placed in the upper area (12 o'clock) and the cocygeal bone (6 o'clock) in the lower area, this is compatible with the cross-section images made by CT. Before removal of the instrument from the anal region, water should be removed from the balloon. In rectosigmoid or sigmoid lesions we have to use the flexible echoendoscope to pass the rectosigmoid junction and to reach the target lesion endoscopically. For examination of the sigmoid region the most important landmarks are the bladder, sacral bone, and major blood vessels, particularly the iliac vessels. After endoscopic visualization of the lesion the balloon or the rectosigmoid lumen can be filled with water in the same way as is used for examination of gastric lesions. For rectal examination the water-filled balloon or water-filled rectum method or both can be used. Whenever possible we prefer to use the water-filled rectum method for adequate visualization of the intraluminal extent of a lesion.

II Endoscopic Ultrasonography of Normal and Pathologic Upper Gastrointestinal Wall Structure

Accurate staging of oesophagogastric malignancy can only be obtained at surgery and after detailed histological examination of the resection specimen. EUS has been reported to be a sensitive diagnostic modality in assessing normal and pathologic gastrointestinal wall structures [1–8]. To further enhance our knowledge regarding the accuracy and limitations of this new diagnostic tool, we investigated prospectively resection specimens and fresh postmortem material of the oesophagus, stomach, and duodenum.

Materials and Methods

Between April 1983 and October 1985 EUS was performed on 10 fresh resection specimens with a normal gastrointestinal wall (Whipple resection), on 5 fresh resection specimens with a benign gastrointestinal lesion, on 10 resection specimens with an oesophagogastric malignancy, and on 5 fresh postmortem specimens.

The resection specimens were investigated in a water bath. The images obtained of the intestinal wall structures were recorded on video tape. Then the investigated areas were marked with metal needles. The various layers were then sequentially removed with micro-dissection under microscopic control and separately examined by EUS. The results of investigations in vivo were compared with those obtained in vitro.

Abnormal areas were marked for subsequent detailed histological examination. A sonographic interpretation was considered correct when clear and precise visualization of the intestinal wall could be obtained which allowed the investigator to draw meaningful conclusions with respect to the intestinal wall structures or the presence of benign or malignant lesions. The studies were performed with an Olympus prototype third- and fourth-generation echoendoscopes, which have been described elsewhere [1–8].

Results

EUS showed that the intestinal wall corresponded to a five layer structure in vitro. Correlation with the various histologic layers was as follows:

The first echogenic structure and the second echo-poor structure bordering on the intestinal lumen correspond to the mucosa, whereas the latter appears to correlate with the muscularis mucosae. This echo-poor structure varied in thickness and was more clearly visualized in the stomach than in the oesophagus.

The third echogenic structure corresponds to the mucosa.

The fourth echopoor structure corresponds to the muscularis propria.

The fifth echogenic structure corresponds to the serosa or adventitia.

The transition between an intact intestinal wall and an area where the muscularis propria and the serosal layer were removed could clearly be demonstrated sonographically (Fig. 1). A corresponding five layer structure was found preoperatively and in vivo (Whipple resection specimen) (Fig. 2). Particularly important was the study of a pancreatic pseudocyst compressing the gastric wall. EUS showed a normal gastric wall structure. Disappearance of the serosal layer and insufficient visualization of the muscularis propria bordering on the pancreatic pseudocyst was explained by similar acoustic impedance of the muscle layer and the cyctic fluid (Fig. 3). EUS revealed a diffuse submucosal hypoechoic structure without penetration into the muscularis propria beyond normal underlying mucosa. This finding was localized in the corpus and antrum of the stomach and confirmed as a benign lesion by autopsy (Fig. 4A). In contrast, EUS allowed visualization of diffuse submucosal infiltration with penetration through the muscularis propria and causing fragmentation of the muscle layer, which was interpreted as highly suggestive of linitis plastica and confirmed by histology of the resection specimen (Fig. 4B). Differentiation between malignant and benign ulcer could be made by follow-up EUS.

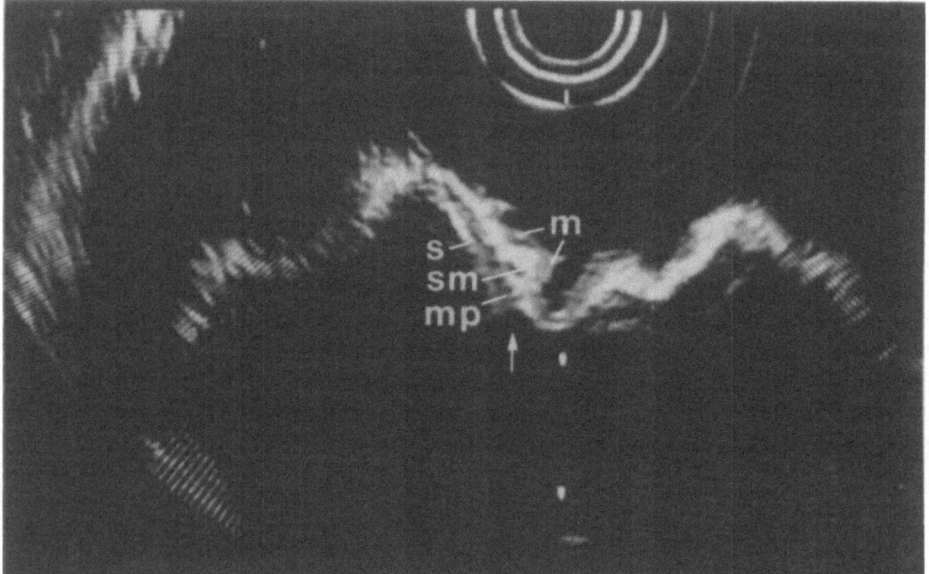

Fig. 1. EUS of stomach resection specimens in vitro showing a five layer structure. The first echogenic and the second echo-poor structure bordering on the transducer correspond to the mucosa *(m)*. The third echogenic structure corresponds to the submucosa *(sm)*. The fourth echo-poor structure corresponds to the muscularis propria *(mp)*. The fifth echo-poor structure corresponds to the serosa *(s)*. The transition between intact wall structure and the area where the muscularis propria and the serosa were removed was clearly visualized *(arrow)*

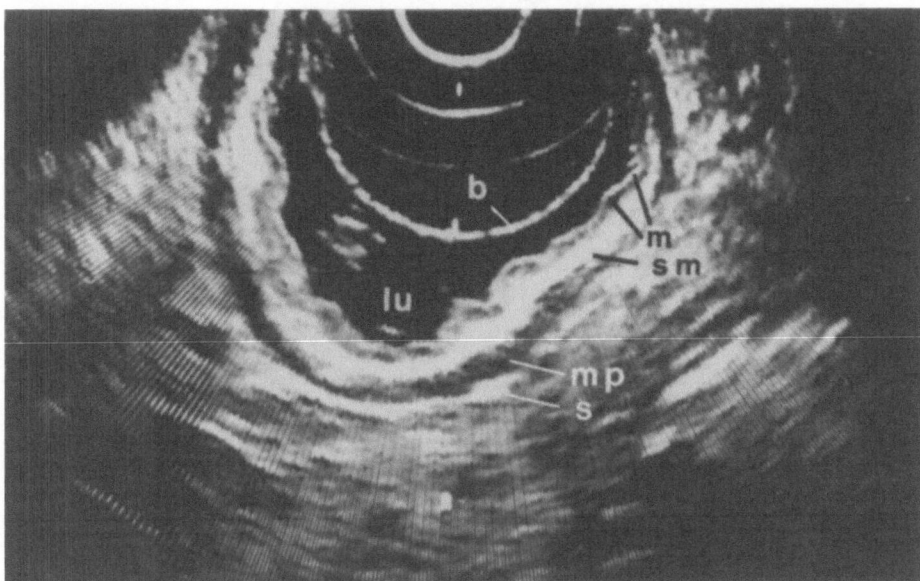

Fig. 2. EUS in vivo showing a corresponding five layer structure of the stomach wall obtained with EUS in vitro. The balloon *(b)* and the stomach lumen *(lu)* are filled with water

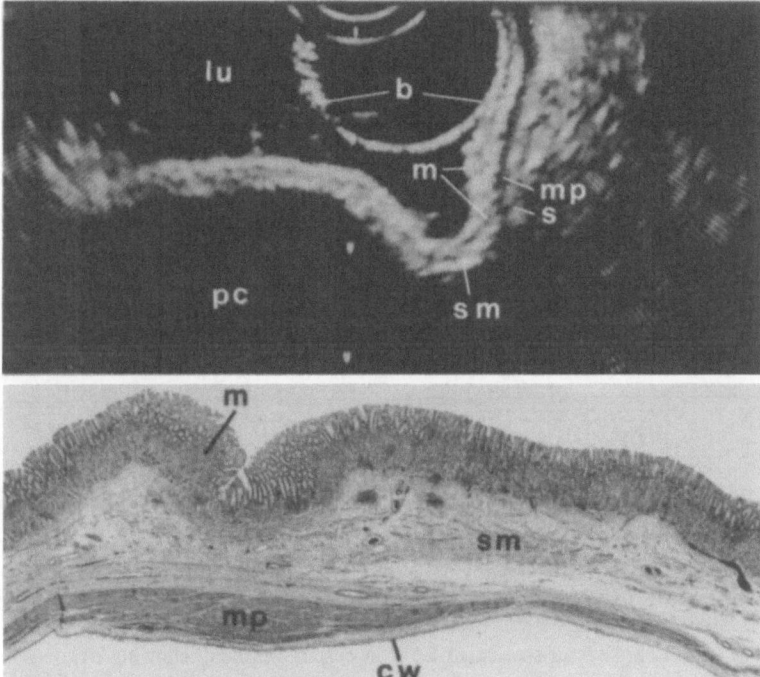

Fig. 3. A EUS of pancreatic pseudocyst *(pc)* compressing the gastric wall. On the right a five layer structure is clearly visualized. Bordering on the pancreatic pseudocyst the muscularis propria and the serosal layer are not clearly seen. **B** Corresponding histology showing normal gastric wall structure with thinning of the muscularis propria and serosal layer and the presence of the cystic wall *(cw)*

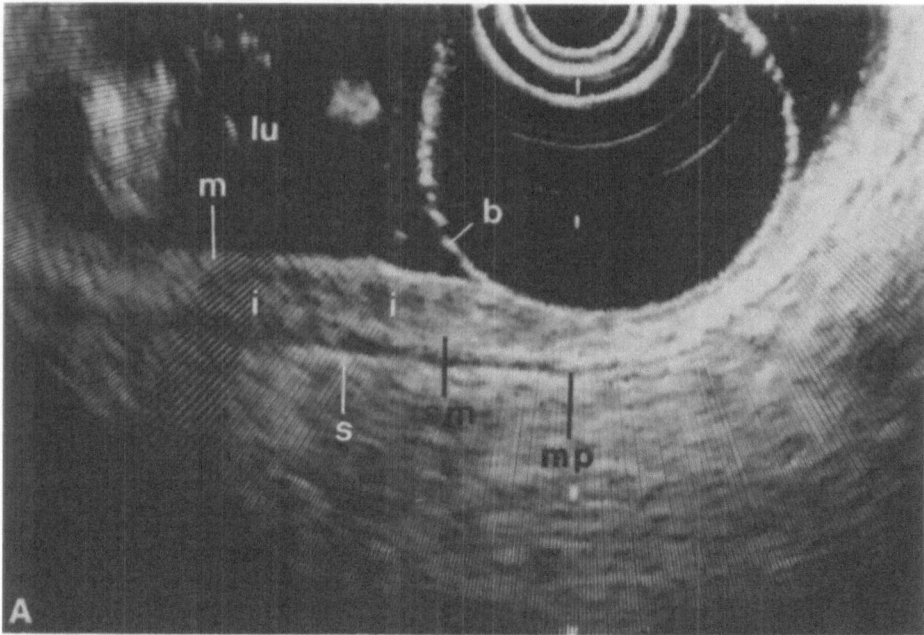

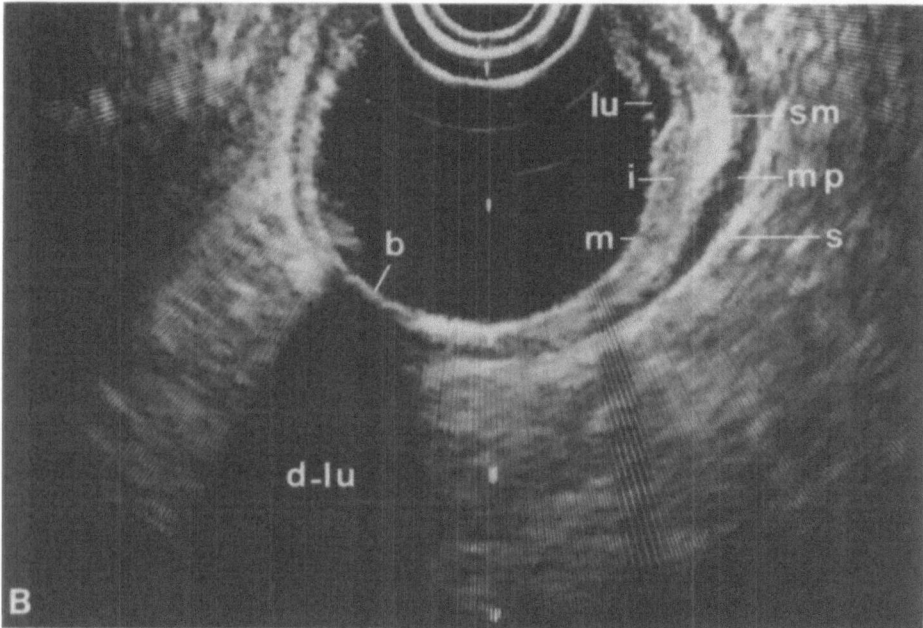

Fig. 4. A Longitudinal section of EUS in corpus ventriculi showing hypoechoic structure in the mucosal and submucosal layer without penetrating into the muscularis propria *(mp)*. **B** Cross-section of EUS in the pyloric region with corresponding hypoechoic structure in the submucosa without penetrating into the muscularis propria. The muscularis propria in the pyloric region appears thicker than in corpus ventriculi. The wall structure on the left appears thinner than on the right because of compression of the water-filled balloon *(b)*

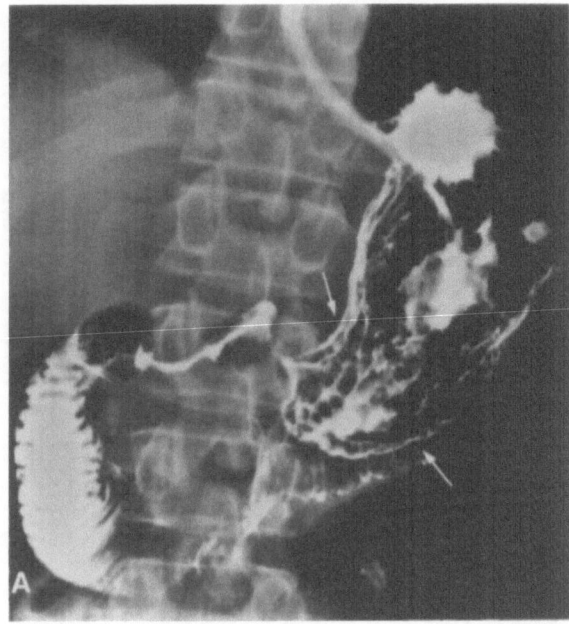

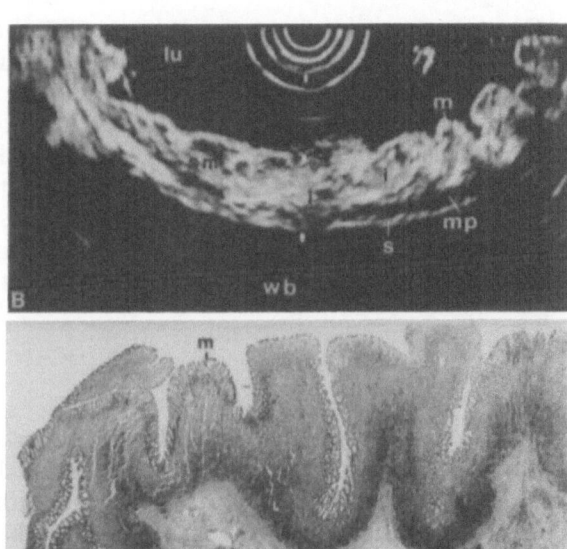

Fig. 5. A Radiology picture showing a double contour *(arrows)* along the lesser and great curvature of the stomach with a narrowing of the pyloric region. **B** EUS in vivo showing diffuse hypoechoic structure *(i)* in the submucosa *(sm)* penetrating into the muscularis propria *(mp)* and into the serosa *(s)*. **C** Corresponding histology showing tumor infiltration *(i)* penetrating the muscularis propria *(mp)*

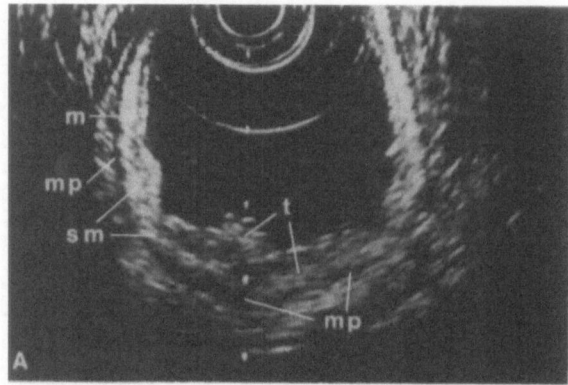

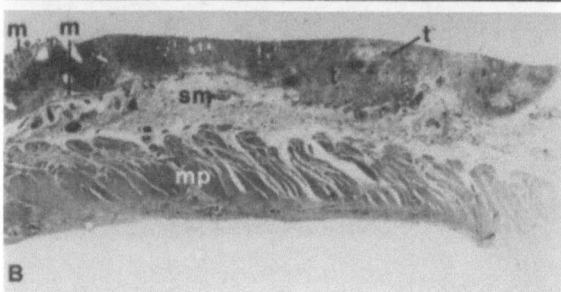

Fig. 6. A EUS in vivo showing hypoechoic structure in the mucosa and submucosa *(t)* without penetrating into the muscularis propria bordering the normal gastric wall structure at both sides. **B** Corresponding histology of the resection specimen showing early gastric cancer *(t)* bordering the normal gastric wall. The resemblance between the EUS image and the corresponding histology is obvious

Disappearance of the intramural abnormality after healing of the ulcer was highly indicative of benignancy contrasting to remaining changes in malignant ulcer. Advanced cancer in the oesophagus and stomach was diagnosed by EUS prior to surgery when a transmurally spreading abnormality was visualized in eight patients and confirmed by histology (Fig. 5). EUS revealed circumscribed infiltration in the mucosa and the submucosa without penetration into the muscularis propria, indicative of early gastric cancer in one of two patients. The finding was confirmed by histology of the resection specimen (Fig. 6). EUS misinterpreted inflammatory infiltration secondary to an ulcer as malignant penetration of early gastric cancer.

Discussion

In this study we have demonstrated that EUS allows accurate visualization of normal and pathologic intestinal wall structures. The normal intestinal wall is usually seen as a five layer structure, which appears to correlate with the histologic wall architecture. Difficulty may arise in clear visualization and in the interpretation of the muscularis mucosae because this muscle layer has a thickness of only approximately 0.4 mm. We feel that EUS enables visualization of such a thin muscle layer based on its axial resolution of approximately 0.2 mm. Moreover, the echo pattern of the muscularis mucosae has features similar to the echo images produced by the muscularis propria. However, this echo-poor structure, which probably correlates with the muscularis mucosae, varies in thickness. Its interpretation is still debatable and needs further evaluation both in vitro and in vivo. More clinically relevant is the clear visualization of the muscularis propria because of its usefulness in distinguishing between a benign and malignant lesion and in differentiating early cancer from advanced cancer in the oesophagus and stomach. A diffuse submucosal abnormality without penetration into the muscularis propria points toward a benign lesion. In contrast, a submucosally spreading lesion with penetration into the muscularis propria is strongly suggestive of linitis plastica. Early cancer can usually be differentiated from advanced cancer when penetration into the muscularis propria is absent. Occasionally a benign lesion with penetration into the muscularis propria secondary to an ulcer may mimic deep infiltration of an early cancer. Differentiation between a benign and a malignant ulcer can readily be made by follow-up investigation. Disappearance of the abnormality after healing of an ulcer is characteristic of its benignancy. Remaining intramural changes are highly suggestive of malignancy.

At present, we feel that a reliable interpretation of the normal and pathologic wall structures is helpful in detecting and staging oesophagogastric malignancy. Further analysis of gastrointestinal wall structures in a larger number of EUS investigations in vivo and in vitro is necessary to enhance the value of this new diagnostic modality.

References

1. Tanaka Y, Yasuda K, Aibe T, Fuji T, Kawai K (1984) Scand J Gastroenterol (suppl 94) 19: 85–90
2. Heyder N, Lutz H, Lux G, Demling L (1984) Scand J Gastroenterol, (suppl 94) 19: 85–90
3. Heyder N, Lutz H, Lux G (1983) Ultraschall, 4: 85–91
4. Strohm WD, Classen M (1984) Ultraschall, 5: 84–93
5. Strohm WD, Kurtz W, Classen M (1984) Scand J Gastroenterol (suppl 94) 19: 60–64
6. Bolondi L, Casanova P, Bertarelli C, Sant V, Caletti G, Labo G (1984) 86: 1031
7. Caletti G, Bolondi L, Labo G (1984) Scand J Gastroenterol (suppl 102) 19: 5–8
8. Tio TL, Tytgat GN (1984) Endoscopy, 4: 220–225

III Endoscopic Ultrasonography in Analysing Peri-Intestinal Lymph Node Abnormality

Transcutaneous ultrasonography is an inadequate investigation for the detection of lymph nodes along the gastrointestinal tract because of the interfering intestinal gas and ribs. Endoscopic ultrasonography (EUS) enables visualization of intestinal abnormalities together with adjacent lymph nodes [1–11]. The purpose of this study was to discuss our experience in detecting and staging lymph node abnormalities in the upper gastrointestinal tract.

Materials and Methods

Between April 1983 and October 1985 EUS was performed on fresh autopsy material, intraoperatively and preoperatively (in vivo), and on corresponding resected specimens (in vitro)., Five autopsy specimens had abnormalities in and adjacent to the gastrointestinal tract. One autopsy specimen showed a bronchus carcinoma penetrating into the oesophagus. Intraoperative EUS examinations were performed in patients suspected of having the Zollinger–Ellison syndrome (one patient), pancreatitis (two patients), pancreatic cancer (five patients), and bronchus carcinoma (one patient). To correlate the EUS findings in vivo (preoperatively) and in vitro, resected specimens of oesophagogastric malignancy (10 patients) and biliopancreatic carcinoma (9 patients) were also investigated.

Methods of Examination

First, we investigated fresh autopsy material to ascertain the shape, size, and internal echo pattern of lymph nodes. Prospectively, lymph nodes detected sonographically were recorded on video tape and then removed for histological examination. The results were compared with the corresponding histological findings.

Second, we performed an intraoperative investigation to detect lymph node abnormalities that could be removed surgically for histological examination.

Third, EUS was performed preoperatively in a series of patients and compared with the EUS findings obtained in the corresponding resected specimens. The results of these investigations were also correlated with subsequent detailed histological examination.

All studies were performed with a 3rd or 4th generation Olympus echoendoscope. All examinations were recorded on videotape, which enabled the investigator to review the sonographic images when necessary.

Results

Investigation of Fresh Postmortem Material

EUS detected round or ellipsoid echo structures that manifested a more hypoechoic pattern than the surrounding tissues. Such structures were confirmed by histology to be lymph nodes in all five specimens. Lymph nodes with an inhomogeneous hypoechoic pattern similar to or more hypoechoic than the echo pattern of the primary lesion, together with sharply demarcated borders, were highly suggestive of malignant lesions as confirmed by histology in all five removed lymph nodes. Lymph nodes with a homogeneous echo pattern, more hyperechoic than the echo pattern of the primary lesion, and with unsharply delineated or pseudopoid boundaries were indicative of benign inflammatory changes, as confirmed by histology.

Intraoperative Investigations

EUS visualized lymph nodes with a homogeneous echo pattern and unsharply demarcated borders, interpreted as non-metastatic lymph nodes and confirmed as benign inflammatory nodes in one patient with chronic pancreatitis. EUS erroneously interpreted round well-demarcated structures with a diameter of 1 cm and with a homogeneous hypoechoic pattern similar to the echo pattern of the spleen as metastasis in a patient with the Zollinger–Ellison syndrome. The structure, however, proved to be an accessory spleen. Three lymph nodes along the splenic artery measuring less than 5 mm were interpreted as non-metastatic, as confirmed by histology.

EUS correctly diagnosed metastatic invasion in 8 of 10 lymph nodes surrounding the primary malignant lesion (Figs. 1, 2). Two micrometastatic lymph nodes measuring less than 2 mm in diameter were erroneously diagnosed as benign lesions.

EUS in vivo (preoperatively) and in vitro (surgical resection specimens) correctly diagnosed malignant infiltration in lymph nodes with a diameter of more than 5 mm adjacent to the primary tumours or the gastric intestinal wall in 8 of 10 resection specimens (Figs. 3, 4). In one resection specimen of pancreatic cancer EUS erroneously diagnosed micrometastasis as reactive inflammation (Fig. 5). EUS also misinterpreted malignant nodes as inflammatory in a patient with polypoid ulcerating advanced gastric cancer because of the hypoechoic pattern and unsharply demarcated borders. These lymph nodes, however, could not accurately be brought into the focus of the beam because of its limited penetration depth.

Discussion

At present, computerized tomography (CT) scan is widely used for detecting and staging lymph node abnormalities in patiens with oesophagogastric and biliopancreatic malignancy [11, 12]. However, CT scan only detects lymph node enlargement and does not enable visualization of internal echoic features that might be helpful to determine the nature of the nodal abnormality [12]. In contrast to conventional ultrasound, EUS provides clear visualization of lymph nodes adjacent to the gastroin-

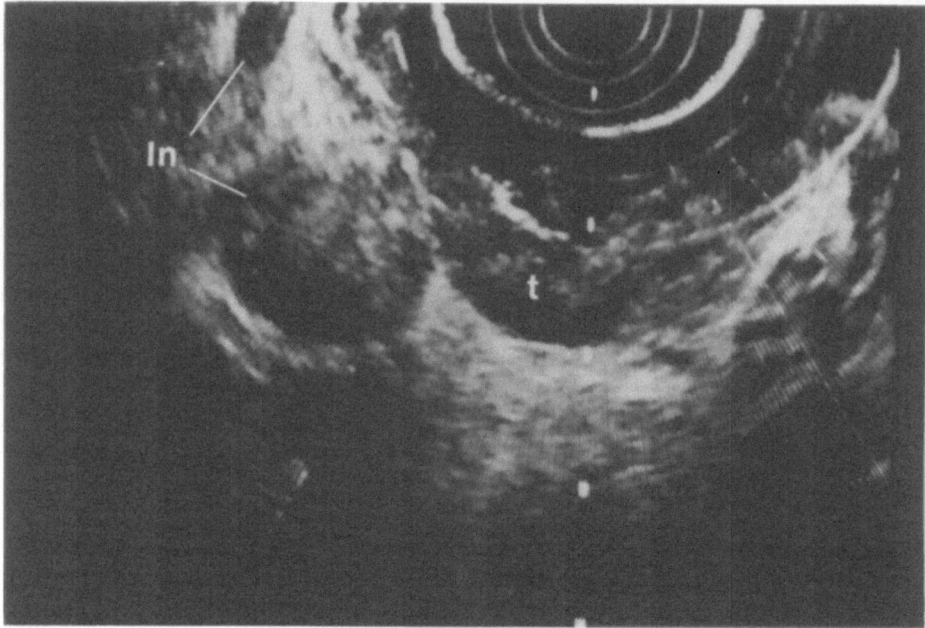

Fig. 1. EUS picture showing two lymph nodes *(ln)* with inhomogeneous hypoechoic echo pattern similar to that of the oesophageal carcinoma *(t)*, revealing sharply demarcated borders highly suggestive of malignancy and confirmed histologically

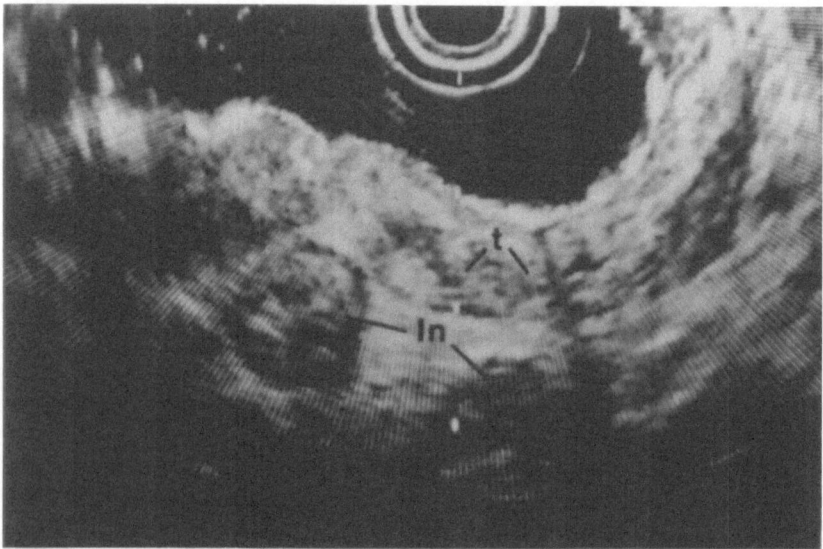

Fig. 2. EUS picture showing a round and ellipsoid lymph node with inhomogeneous hypoechoic structure more hypoechoic than the gastric carcinoma, revealing sharply delineated boundaries proven to be malignant by histology

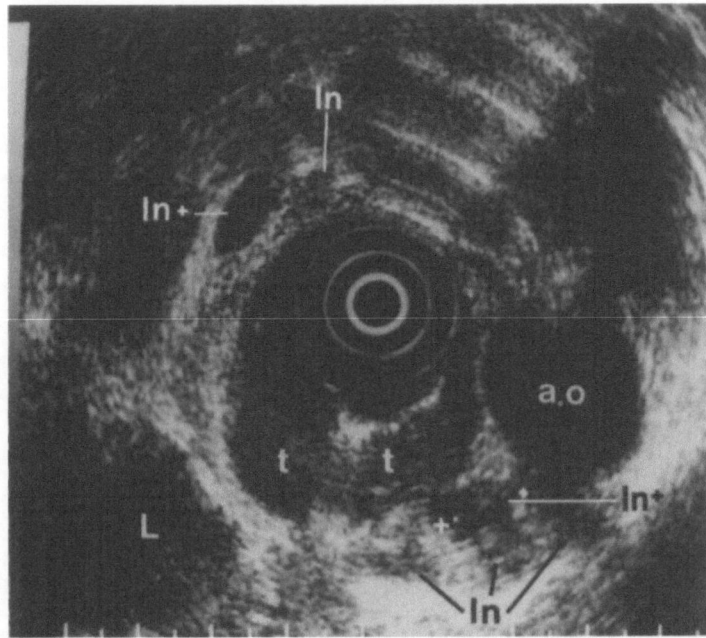

Fig. 3. EUS picture showing ellipsoid lymph nodes *(ln⁺)* with inhomogeneous echo pattern similar to that of the oesophageal carcinoma, revealing sharply delineated borders proven to be malignant histologically, contrasting with the hyperechoic homogeneous echo structure with unsharply delineated boundaries of benign lymph nodes *(ln)*

testinal tract or biliopancreatic system because of the high resolution of this new diagnostic modality. Such lymph nodes are readily recognized on the basis of their more hypoechoic pattern as compared with the echo pattern of the surrounding tissues. It appears from our studies that lymph nodes with an inhomogeneous hypoechoic structure similar to or more hypoechoic than the echo pattern of the primary lesion together with sharply demarcated borders are highly suggestive of malignancy. In contrast, lymph nodes with a hyperechoic homogeneous echo pattern as compared with the primary lesion together with unsharply delineated or pseudopoid boundaries are often indicative of reactive inflammatory changes. Difficulties may arise when lymph nodes cannot accurately be brought into the focus of the beam or when the diameter of the nodes is smaller than 2 mm. Moreover, micrometastasis often cannot be differentiated from inflammatory changes.

Although the number of prospective investigations in vivo and in vitro is still limited, we believe that EUS will become an important diagnostic tool in detecting and staging lymph node abnormality. Further studies in preoperative staging of oesophagogastric malignancy and biliopancreatic carcinoma and prospective ultrasonic evaluation of resection specimens may enhance our knowledge in the interpretation of lymph node abnormalities.

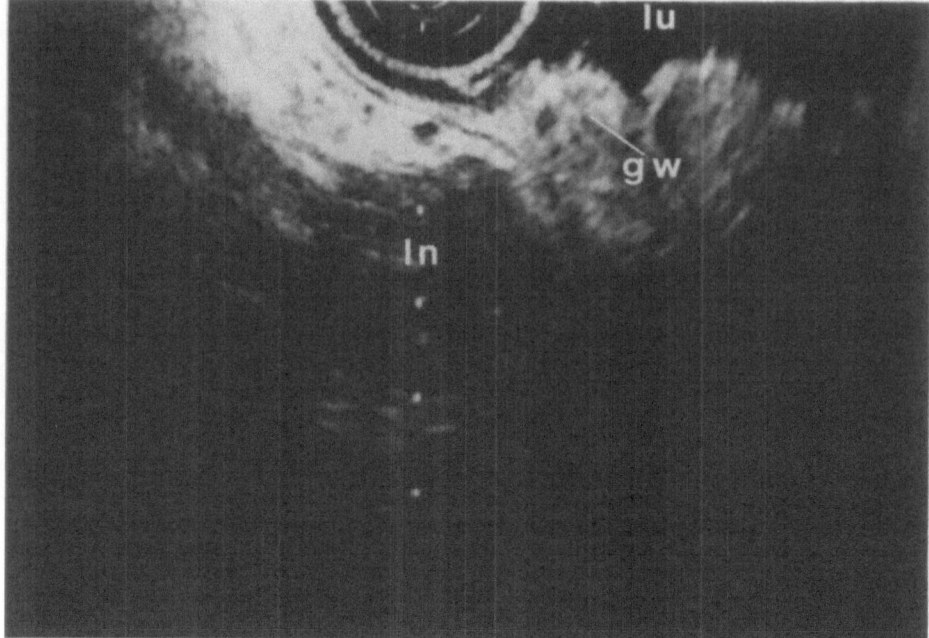

a

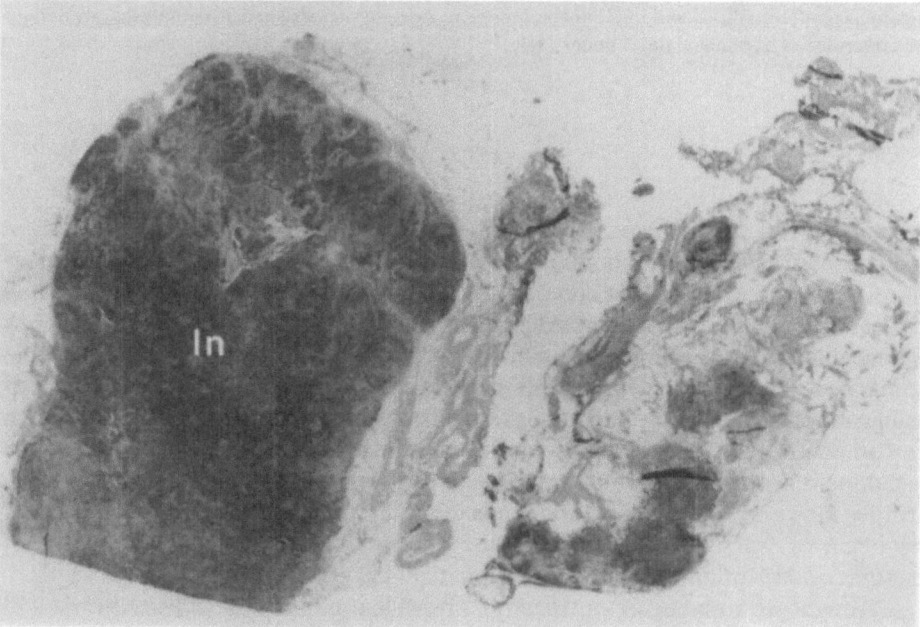

b

Fig. 4. AEUS picture showing hypoechoic inhomogeneous echo structure adjacent to the gastric wall, revealing nodular sharply demarcated boundaries. **B** Corresponding histology of the lymph node proven to be malignantly infiltrated. The correspondence between EUS image and correspondence between EUS image and corresponding histology is readily appreciated

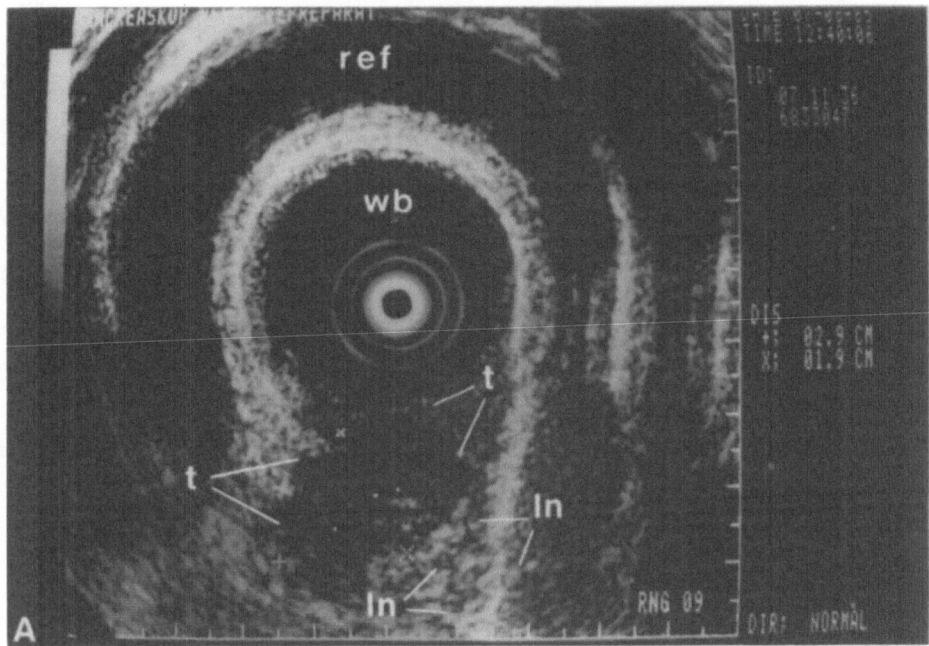

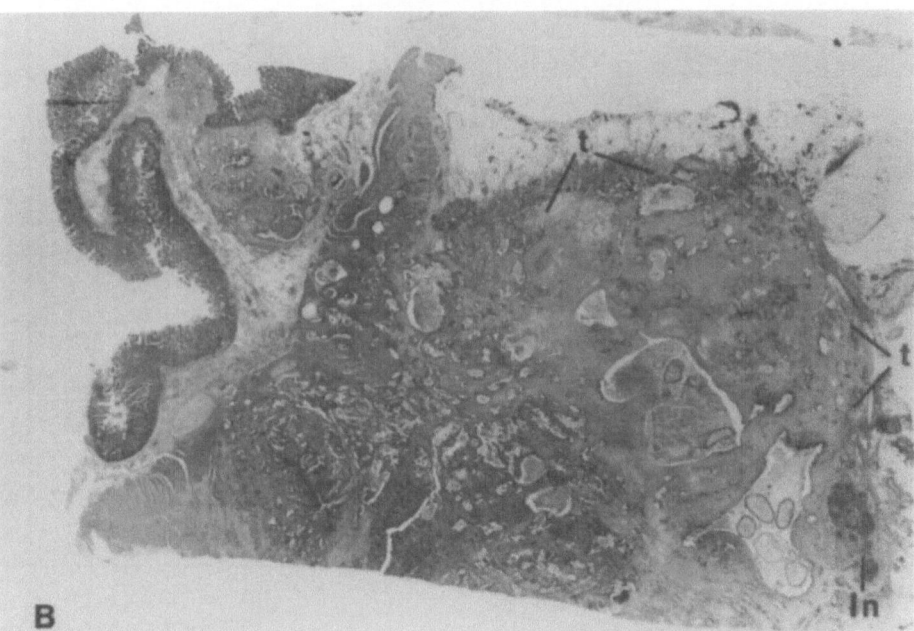

Fig. 5. AEUS picture of the resection specimen of a pancreatic cancer (Whipple resection), showing quite small lymph nodes with a diameter between 1 and 2 mm, revealing hyperechoic structures with unsharply demarcated or pseudopoid boundaries adjacent to pancreatic cancer *(t)* indicative of benignancy. **B** Corresponding histology of pancreatic cancer *(t)* with micrometastasis in lymph nodes. The correspondence of the tumour and lymph nodes in size and configuration are obvious

References

1. Di Magno EP, Regan PT, Clain JE, James EM, Buxtm JM (1982) Gastroenterology 83: 824–829
2. Lux G, Heyder N, Demling L (1982) Endoscopy 4: 220–225
3. Heyder N, Lutz H, Lux G (1983) Ultraschall, 85–91
4. Tio TL, Tytgat GNJ (1984) Endoscopy 4: 220–225
5. Classen M, Strohm WD, Kurtz W (1984) Scand Gastroenterol (suppl 94) 19: 77–84
6. Fukuda M, Nakano Y, Saito K, Hirata K, Terada S, Urushizaki I (1984) Scand J Gastroenterol (suppl 94) 19: 65–76
7. Bolondi L, Casanova P, Bertarelli C, Santi V, Caletti G, Labò G (1984) Gastroenterology [Abstract] 86: 1031
8. Caletti G, Bolondi L, Labò G (1984) Scand J Gastroenterol (suppl 102) 19: 5–8
9. Strohm WD, Kurtz W, Classen M (1984) Scand J Gastroenterol (suppl 94) 19: 60–64
10. Yasuda K, Tanaka Y, Fujimoto S, Nakajima M, Kawai K (1984) Scand J Gastroenterol (suppl 102) 19: 9–17
11. Wittenberg J, Ferrucci JT (1978) Gastroenterology 74: 287–293
12. Stephens D, Sheedy PF, Hatery RH (1983) In: Greenberg M (ed) Essentials of body computed tomography. Saunders, Philadelphia, 212–227

IV The Role of Endoscopic Ultrasonography in Assessing Local Resectability of Oesophagogastric Malignancies

Prediction of the resectability of GI tumours before surgery is still quite difficult despite diagnostic advances [1–5]. Endoscopic ultrasonography (EUS) may provide accurate detection and staging of oesophagogastric malignancy because of its ability to visualize both the intramural and extramural extent of the lesion and any adjacent lymph node involvement [6–13]. To determine the accuracy and limitations of this new diagnostic modality, we prospectively investigated a consecutive series of patients with upper intestinal malignancy and compared the EUS findings with those obtained at surgery and at histological examination of the resected specimen.

Materials and Methods

Between April 1983 and October 1985, preoperative EUS was performed in 62 patients who all underwent surgery for oesophagogastric malignancy. There were 26 patients with oesophageal carcinoma, 17 men and 9 women, with an age ranging from 44 to 80 years. There were 36 patients with gastric carcinoma, 31 men and 5 women, with an age ranging from 27 to 82 years. These patients were divided into three groups, to assess the accuracy of EUS in predicting resectability before surgery.

Group 1. Local resectability was diagnosed when EUS found a clearly demarcated intramural lesion without deep infiltration into the surrounding tissues and without or with loco-regional but not distant lymph node abnormality.

Group 2. Palliative resectability was diagnosed when distant lymph node abnormality was detected in the presence of a clearly demarcated intramural lesion without deep infiltration into the surrounding tissues.

Group 3. Local non-resectability was diagnosed when deep infiltration of the tumour into the surrounding tissues and/or organs was found, usually combined with multiple adjacent lymph nodes, with suspicion of metastatic spread.

Ten fresh resection specimens were investigated, to correlate the findings of EUS in vivo (preoperative EUS) and in vitro (EUS of resected specimen).

The results of all EUS examinations were correlated with those obtained at surgical exploration and histological examination of the resected specimens.

The endoscopic ultrasonographic studies were performed with a prototype 3rd generation GF-UM1 Olympus echoendoscope which has been described elsewhere

[6–13]. In five patients a 4th generation GF-UM2 Olympus echoendoscope with 360° sector scan was used, the technical data of which are comparable to those of the 3rd generation echoendoscope. The method and the documentation of the examination has been described elsewhere [6–13].

Complications were not encountered in this study.

Results

Table 1 summarizes the results of EUS compared with surgical exploration, in assessing local, palliative, and non-resectability of oesophageal malignancy.

Table 1. Comparison of results of EUS and surgery in assessing local resectability, palliative resectability, and local non-resectability of oesophageal malignancy

N	Local resectability (EUS/surg.)	Palliative resectability (EUS/surg.)	Local non-resectability (EUS/surg.)
26	5/6	11/13	6/7

Local resectability was correctly diagnosed with EUS in five of six patients because a clearly demarcated intramural mass without deep infiltration into the surrounding tissues and without (three patients) and with (two patients) loco-regional lymph node abnormality was found, which was confirmed at surgery and by histology of the resection specimens (Fig. 1). Of the six patients EUS misinterpreted chronic inflammatory action as malignant infiltration in a patient who had a surgical hiatal hernia repair.

Palliative resection was accurately predicted by EUS in 11 of 13 patients because abnormal distant lymph nodes were detected together with a clearly demarcated tumour mass without deep infiltration into the surrounding tissues, which was confirmed at surgery and by histology (Fig. 2). In 2 of 13 patients very small lymph nodes with an abnormal echopattern were misinterpreted as "reactive inflammation", but histology showed micrometastasis.

EUS clearly visualized deep malignant infiltration into the pericardium (two patients), the bronchus (two), major blood vessels (one), and adjacent liver (one) and thereby accurately predicted the local non-resectability in six of seven patients (Figs. 3–5). These findings were confirmed at surgery, and the tumours were proven to be locally non-resectable. EUS failed to document local non-resectability in one of seven patients because the stenosis could not be passed with the echoendoscope.

Table 2 summarizes the results of EUS compared with surgical exploration in assessing local, palliative, and local non-resectability of stomach malignancy.

EUS accurately detected a clearly demarcated infiltrative growth in 9 of 11 patients (Fig. 6). Loco-regional but not distant lymph node abormalities indicative of malignancy were found in 3 of 11 patients. The prediction of local resectability and loco-

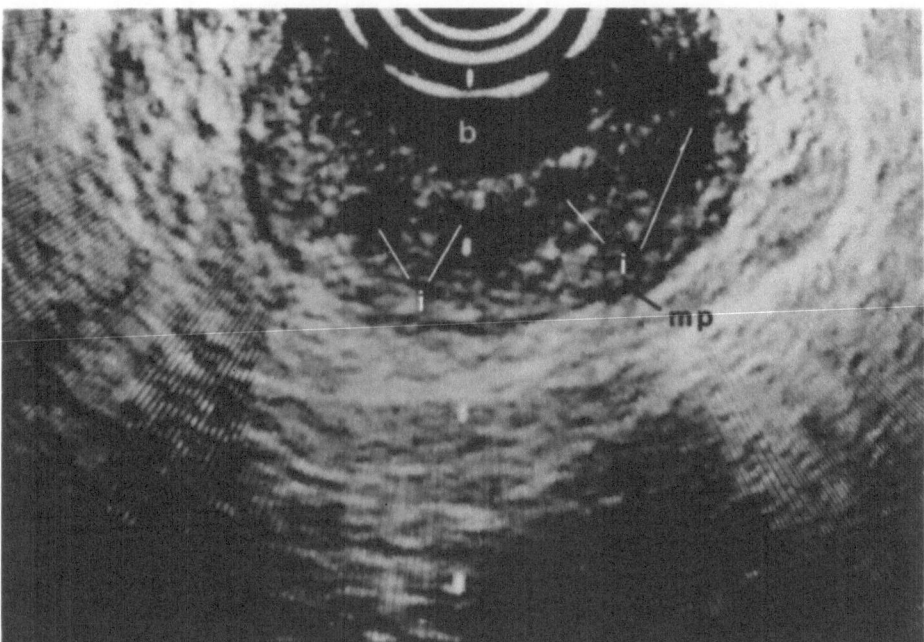

Fig. 1. EUS of intramural hypoechoic infiltration (*i*) bordering on the water-filled balloon
(b) without penetration into the muscularis propria *(mp)*

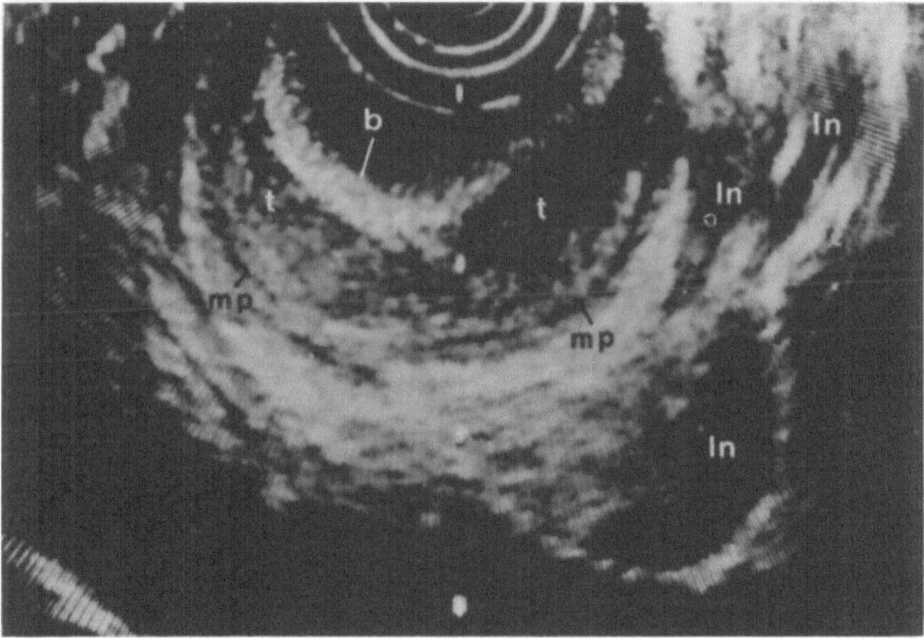

Fig. 2. EUS of transmural infiltration (*t*) with penetration into the muscularis propria *(mp)* and
involved lymph nodes *(ln)*

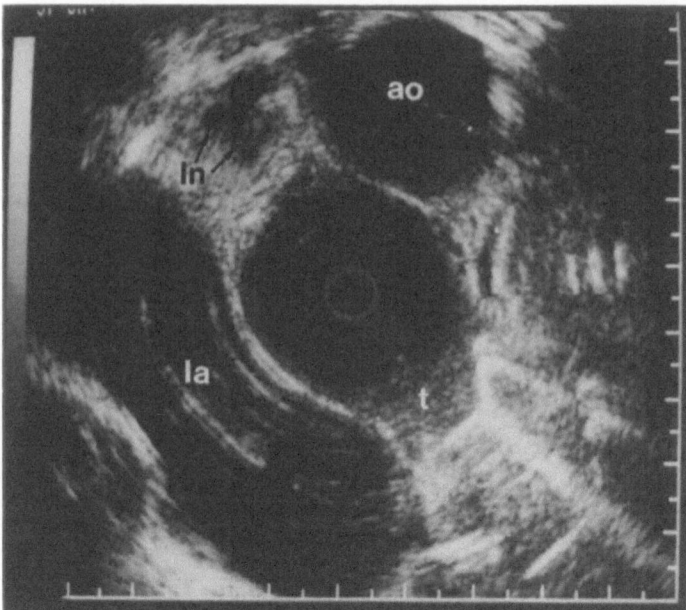

Fig. 3. EUS of transmural infiltrating tumour (*t*) with infiltration into the pericardium of the left atrium (*la*) and paraortic (*ao*) lymph node involvement (*ln*), by means of echoendoscope with 360° sector

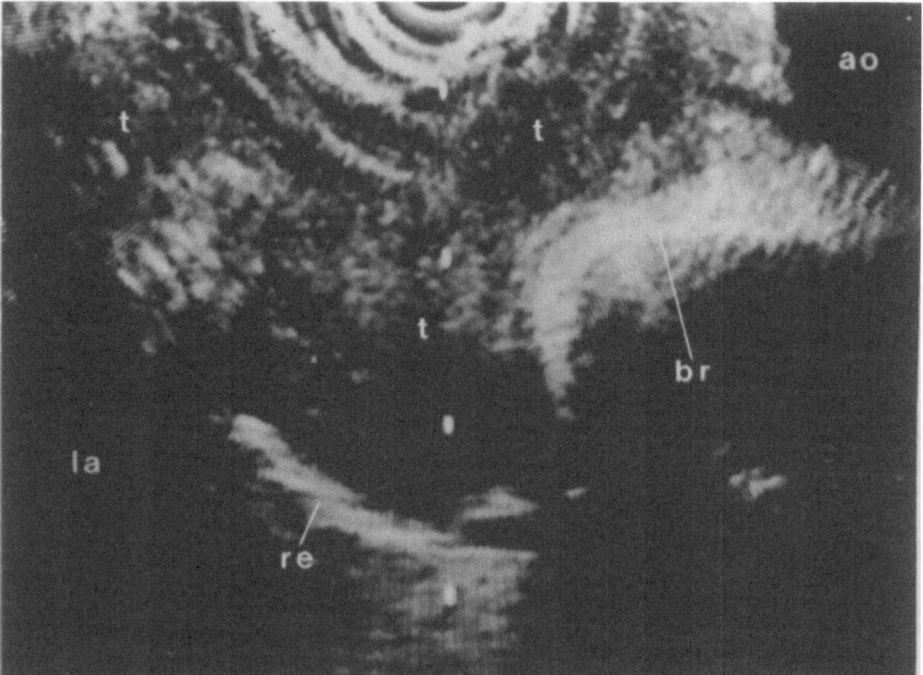

Fig. 4. EUS of tumour (*t*) with deep infiltration into the surrounding tissues, particularly to the bronchus (*br*)

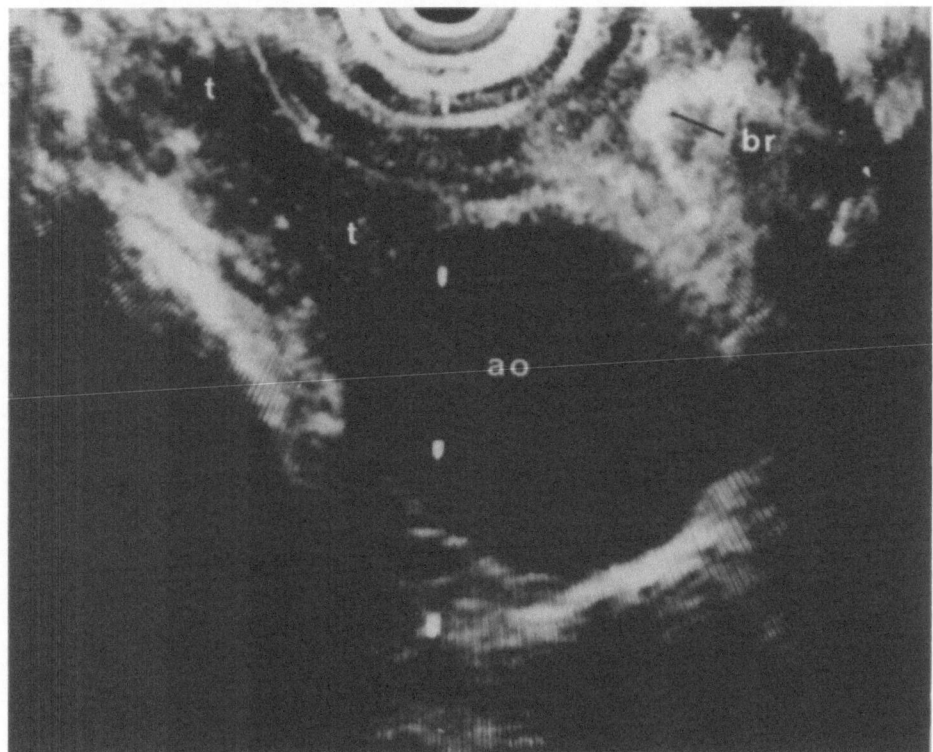

Fig. 5. EUS of tumour (*t*) infiltrating into the aorta

Table 2. Comparison of results of EUS and surgery in assessing local, palliative, and local non-resectability of stomach malignancy

N	Local resectability (EUS/surg.)	Palliative resectability (EUS/surg.)	Local non-resectability (EUS/surg.)
36	9/11	13/15	8/10

regional lymph node metastasis was confirmed at surgery and by histology. EUS misdiagnosed metastatic lymph nodes surrounding a polypoid ulcerative lesion as reactive inflammaction in one of four patients with lymph node metastasis.

A correct prediction of palliative resection was made by EUS in 13 of 15 patients on the basis of the presence of distant malignant lymph nodes in the presence of a sharply defined tumour without deep infiltration into the surrounding tissues (Fig. 7). Pseudoinvasion, mimicking malignant infiltration into the adjacent liver, secondary to compression of the lesion by the water-filled balloon, was found with EUS in one patient (Fig. 8).

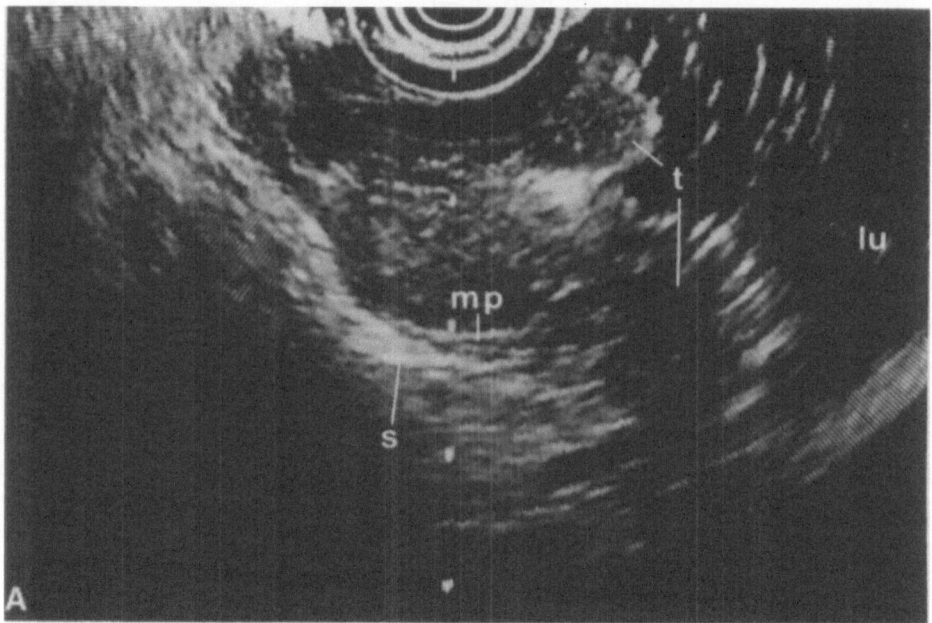

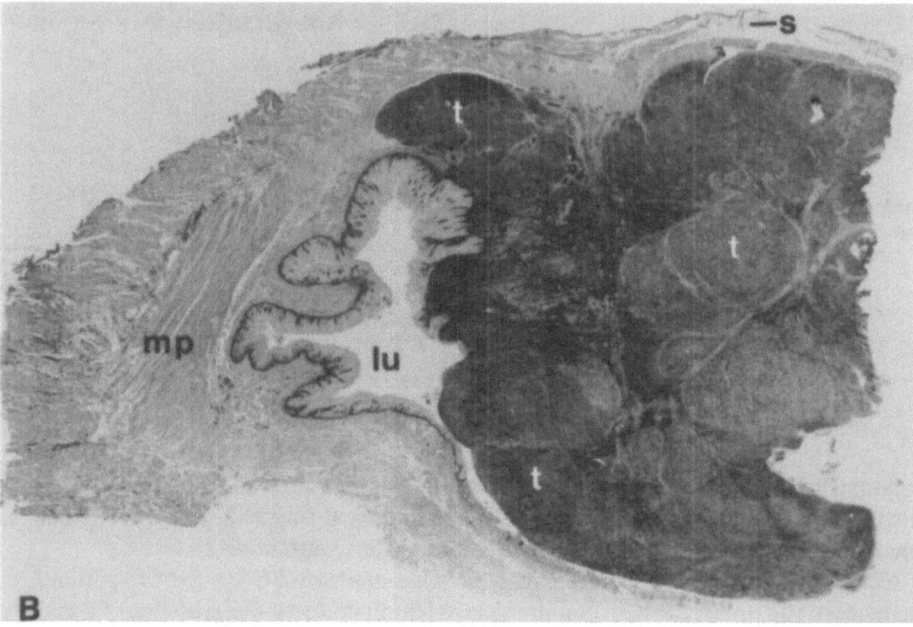

Fig. 6. A EUS of polypoid exophytic tumour (*t*) of the fundus infiltrating the muscularis propria (*mp*), obtained after filling the lumen (*lu*) with water. **B** Corresponding histology showing an exophytic adenocarcinoma penetrating the muscularis propria. The resemblance between the EUS picture and the corresponding histology is obvious

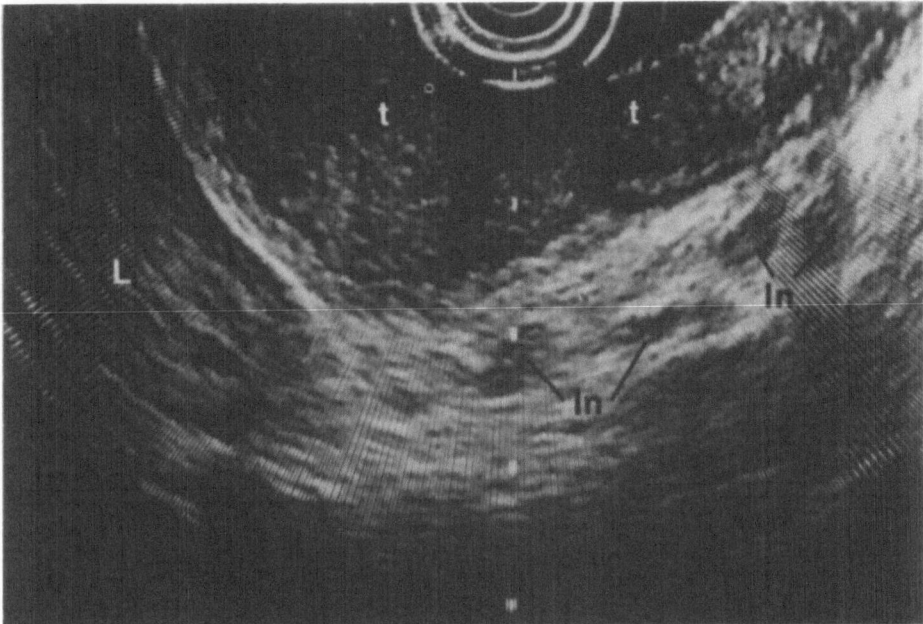

Fig. 7. EUS of transmural gastric tumour (*t*) bordering the left lobe of the liver (*L*) with multiple involved lymph nodes (*ln*) along the small curvature of the stomach

EUS clearly showed deep infiltration into the pancreas, along the small curvature of the stomach into the liver, the portal vein (hepatoduodenal ligament) and large blood vessels in 8 of 10 patients, which was confirmed as locally non-resectable carcinoma at surgery (Figs. 9, 10). EUS failed to document penetration into the surrounding tissues or organs in 2 of 10 patients because of the inability of the echoendoscope to pass the stenosis.

Discussion

EUS appears to be an accurate diagnostic procedure in the preoperative assessment of resectability of oesophagogastric malignancy because of its detailed visualisation of the depth of penetration into the surrounding tissues and/or organs. Although not studied in this analysis, we have the impression that EUS will prove to be superior to any other diagnostic modality in staging malignancy and in assessing resectability. The detection of a clearly defined lesion infiltrating the intestinal wall without or with loco-regional lymph node involvement is shown to indicate local resectability of malignancy. Distant lymph node involvement – that is, nodes with irregular hypoechoic echopattern and sharply demarcated borders – in the presence of a locally resectable tumour strongly indicates the palliative nature of the resection. Deep infiltration of the malignancy into the surrounding tissues and/or organs is strongly suggestive of

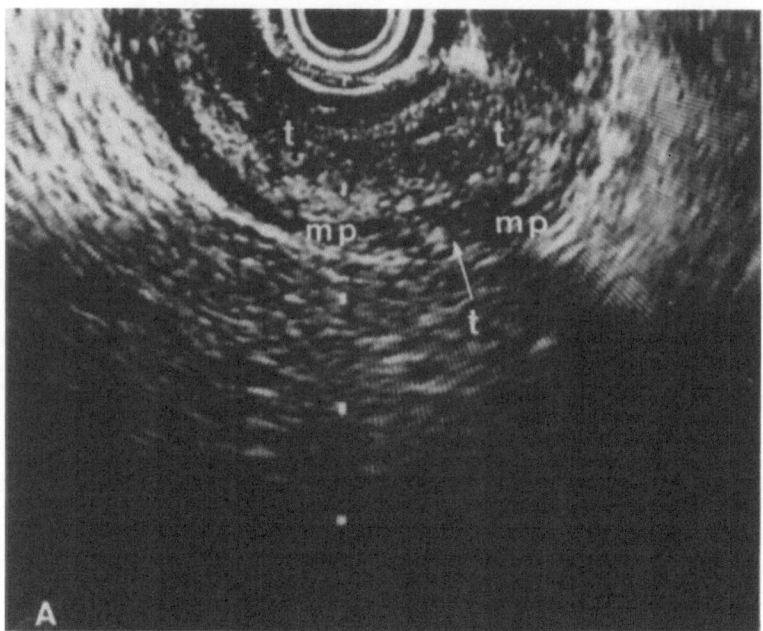

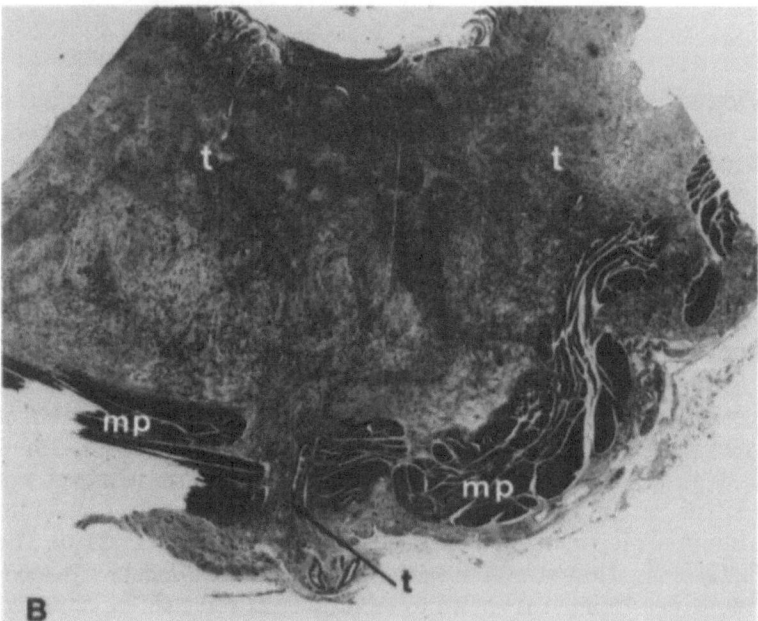

Fig. 8. A EUS of transmural tumour (*t*) penetrating the muscularis propria (*mp*) with dubious borders to the liver. **B** Histological picture of the tumour with penetration through the muscularis propria into the serosa. The correspondence between the EUS image and the histology of the resection specimen is easily seen

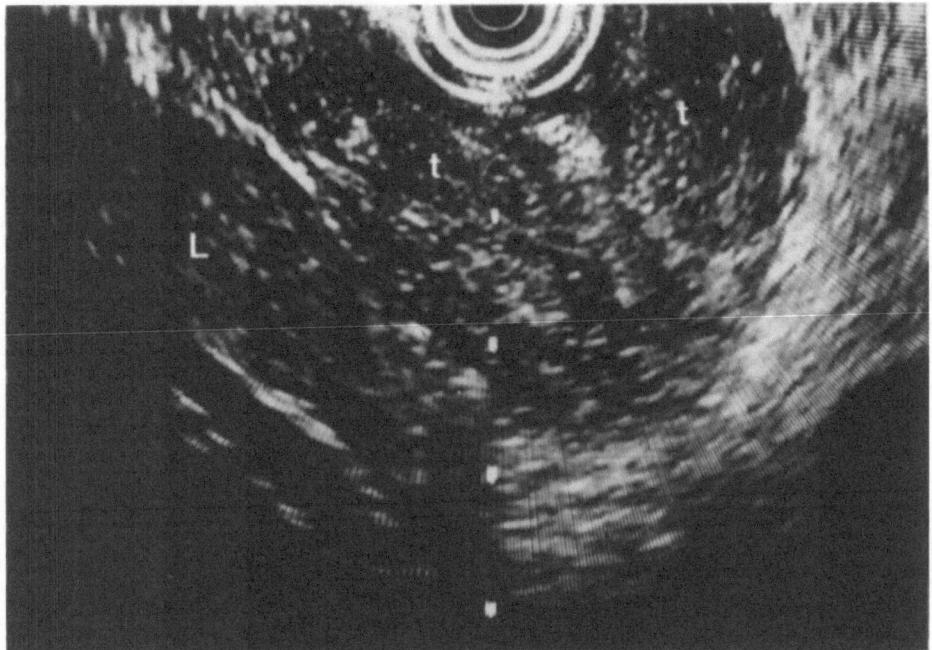

Fig. 9. EUS of extensive tumour (*t*) infiltrating the adjacent liver (*L*)

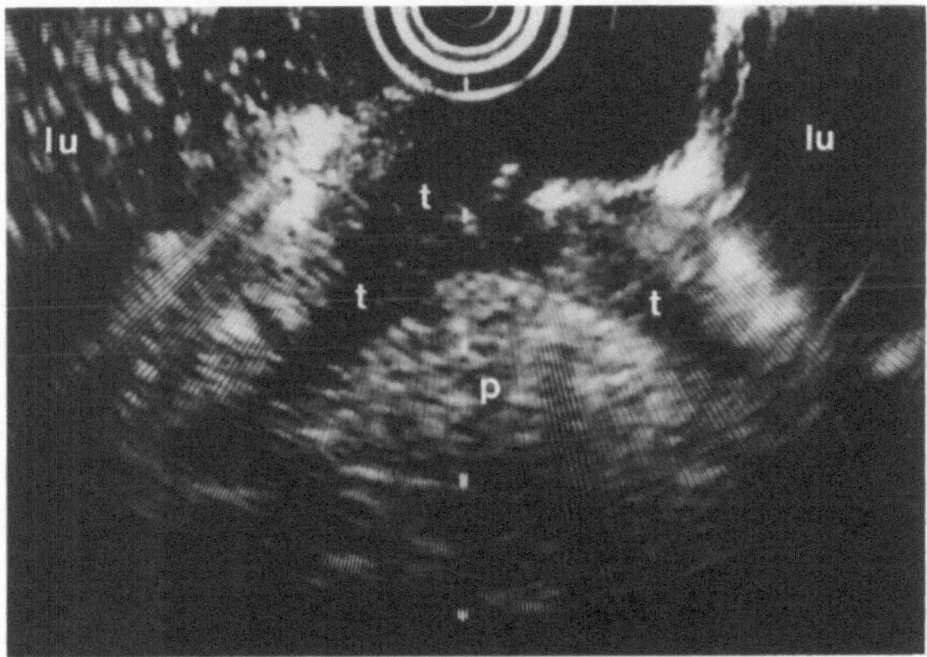

Fig. 10. EUS of deep infiltration (*t*) into the pancreas (*p*), proven to be inoperable at surgery

local non-resectability. Occasionally, difficulty may arise in differentiating very small metastatic lymph node involvement from reactive inflammatory changes. Furthermore, pseudoinvasion due to compression of the lesion by the water-filled balloon may mimic deep penetration of malignancy into the surrounding tissues. Removal of the water from the balloon should be helpful in assessing the true depth of invasion, particularly in stenotic areas.

The side-viewing optics of the echoendoscope do not enable detailed endoscopic study in the upper GI tract. It is therefore desirable that the operator obtains endoscopic information before the EUS investigation. Because the focus of the ultrasonic beam is at 35 mm, the lesions must be brought into focus to achieve optimal ultrasonographic resolution. This is not always possible, particularly in the presence of stenotic lesions. Technical improvements, reducing the lenght of the rigid tip and allowing cytologic sonographically guided puncture, may further enhance the value of EUS.

References

1. Kressel HY, Callen PW, Montague JP, Korobkin M (1978) Radiology 129: 451–455
2. Lee KR, Levine E, Moffat RE, Bigongiari LR, Hermreck AS (1979) Radiology 133: 151–155
3. Parienty RA, Smolarski N, Pradel J, Ducellier R, Lubrano JM (1979) J Comput Assist 3: 615–619
4. Köster O, Harder T (1982) Fortschr Rontgenstr 137: 727–729
5. Crone-Münzbrock W, Brockmann WP (1982) Fortschr Rontgenstr 139: 676–680
6. Caletti G, Bolondi L (1983) [Abstract] Gastroenterology 84: 1366
7. Tio TL, Tytgat GN (1984) Endoscopy 4: 220–225
8. Caletti G, Bolondi L, Labò G (1984) Scand J Gastroenterol (suppl 102) 19: 5–8
9. Heyder N, Lutz H, Lux G (1983) Ultraschall 4: 85–91
10. Strohm WD, Classen M (1984) Ultraschall 5: 84–93
11. Lux G, Heyder N, Demling L (1982) Endoscopy 4: 220–225
12. Fukuda M, Nakano Y, Saito K, Hirata K, Terada S, Urushizaki I (1984) Scand J Gastroenterol (suppl 94) 19: 65–76
13. Strohm WD, Kurtz W, Classen M (1984) Scand J Gastroenterol (suppl 94) 19: 60–64

V Endoscopic Ultrasonography in Staging Local Resectability of Pancreatic and Periampullary Malignancy

Pancreatic cancer is still detected at a rather late stage, and 80–90% of the cases are incurable despite major advances in diagnostic imaging techniques [1, 2]. In general, the resectability rate of pancreatic cancer is less than that of periampullary carcinoma [3, 4]. Endoscopic ultrasonography (EUS) enables detailed visualization of the pancreas, the pancreatic duct, and its surrounding structures without being hindered by air or obesity [5–12].

The purpose of this study was to ascertain prospectively the accuracy and limitations of EUS in staging pancreatic and periampullary malignancy. Particular attention was given to the possibility of predicting resectability before surgery.

Materials and Methods

Between April 1983 and October 1985 EUS was performed in 70 patients with pancreatic cancer and in 15 patients with periampullary malignancy. For this analysis, we included only patients in whom the final diagnosis and staging were carried out at surgery. The patients fell into two groups. The first group consisted of 14 patients with pancreatic cancer. There were nine men and five women; their ages ranged from 42 to 73 years, with an average of 58 years. The second group consisted of nine patients with periampullary carcinoma. There were six men and three women; their ages ranged from 51 to 79 years, with an average of 59 years.

Five fresh surgical resection specimens were investigated both in vivo and in vitro, to compare the results of EUS in vivo (pre- or intra-operative EUS) with EUS in vitro. Intraoperative EUS was performed in five patients with pancreatic cancer. The results of EUS were compared with the findings obtained at surgical exploration and at detailed histological examination of the resection specimens.

The endoscopic ultrasonographic studies were performed with a prototype 3rd generation GF-UM1 Olympus echoendoscope, which has been described elsewhere [7–12]. In four patients a 4th generation Olympus GF-UM2 echoendoscope with a 360° sector scan with the capability of recording the patient data and of measuring the extent of the lesion was used. The gastric lumen was filled with deaerated (boiled) water to facilitate visualization of the body and tail of the pancreas. The head of the pancreas could usually not be examined from the distal part of the stomach. The ampullary region and the uncinate process had to be investigated from the duodenum. Rapid filling of the duodenal lumen with water enabled visualization of polypoid lesions in the periampullary region. Complications were not encountered in the study.

To enable the assessment of the accuracy of EUS staging, the lesions were prospectively subdivided into three categories.

A lesion was considered to be locally resectable when EUS visualized a clearly demarcated malignant growth without evidence of suspicious lymph nodes around the mass.

A lesion was considered to be palliatively resectable when EUS visualized a well-demarcated mass but in the presence of multiple distant lymph nodes, which were suggestive of metastatic spread.

A lesion was considered non-resectable when EUS visualized a malignant growth revealing deep infiltration around and into the adjacent major blood vessel (such as mesenteric artery, coeliac trunk, aorta) and adjacent structures or metastatic spread to the adjacent liver, usually in the presence of metastatic lymph node involvement.

Results

Table 1 summarizes the results of EUS compared with surgical exploration in assessing local and palliative resectability and non-resectability of pancreatic cancer.

Table 1. Comparison of EUS and surgery in assessing local and palliative resectability and non-resectability of pancreatic cancer

n	Local resectability (EUS/surg.)	Palliative resectability (EUS/surg.)	Local non-resectability (EUS/surg.)
14	3/3	4/5	5/6

In three patients EUS detected a sharply delineated tumour, localized twice in the pancreatic duct and once in the intra-ampullary common bile duct without evidence of lymph node involvement, which was confirmed by detailed histological examination of the resection specimens (Fig. 1).

A clearly delineated, round or polycyclic tumour mass with a characteristic hypoechoic echo pattern when compared with the surrounding pancreas parenchyma, with evidence of lymph node involvement, was seen by EUS in four of five patients (Fig. 2).

Compression of the pancreatic duct and/or prestenotic dilatation secondary to the compressing tumour could readily be visualized (Fig. 3). In these patients EUS predicted that the resectability should be on the basis of the presence of multiple lymph nodes, although the tumour was considered locally resectable, which was confirmed histologically. In one patient, the suspicion of lymph node metastasis at EUS proved to be incorrect. In five of six patients, non-resectability was suggested by EUS because of deep infiltration of the tumour into or around major blood vessels (Fig. 4) and/or organs (mesenteric artery, coeliac trunk, aorta, or liver metastasis) EUS enabled accurate delineation of the extent of the tumour mass, of the presence of

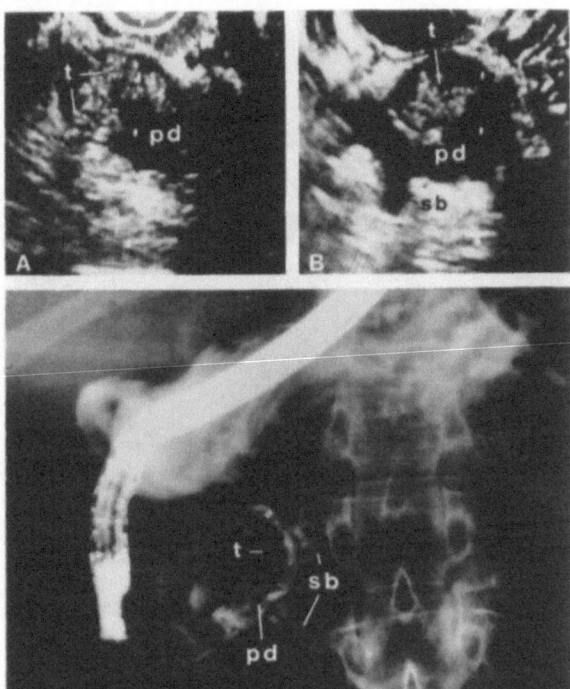

Fig. 1. A EUS picture showing clearly an intraductal tumour *(t)* originating from pancreatic duct *(arrow)* and dilatation of the pancreatic duct *(pd)*. **B** Another cross-section of EUS showing dilatation of pancreatic duct and side branches *(sb)* together with visualization of an intraductal tumour mass *(t)* **C** Dilatation of pancreatic duct and side brances *(sb)* suggestive of malignant tumour *(t)* in the head of the pancreas found on ERCP. **D** Corresponding macroscopic picture of resected specimen showing multilocated intraductal carcinomas *(t)* in an extremely dilated pancreatic duct *(pd)*

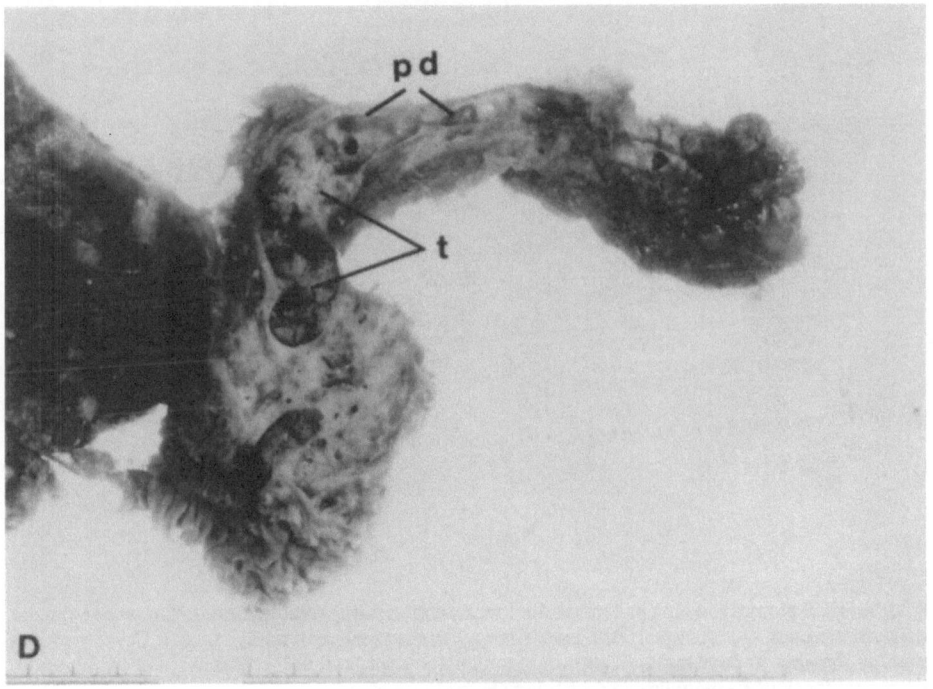

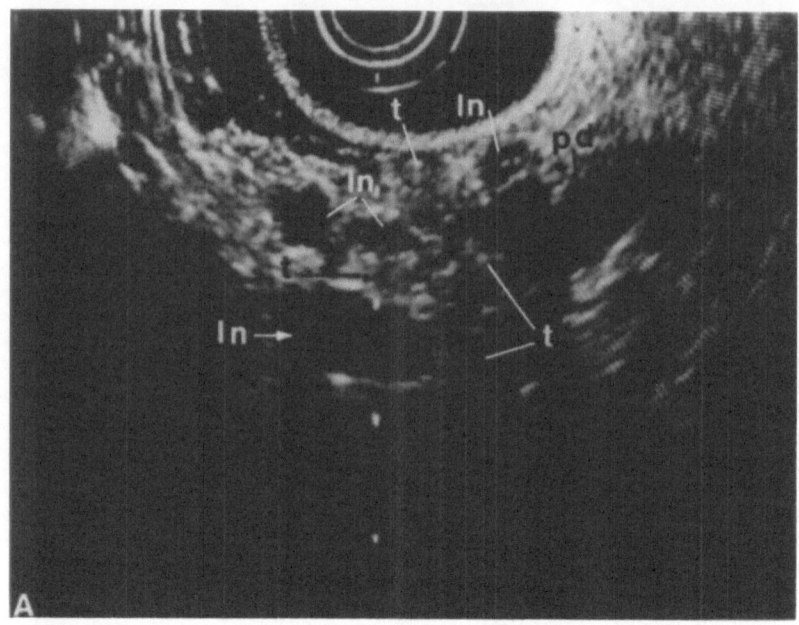

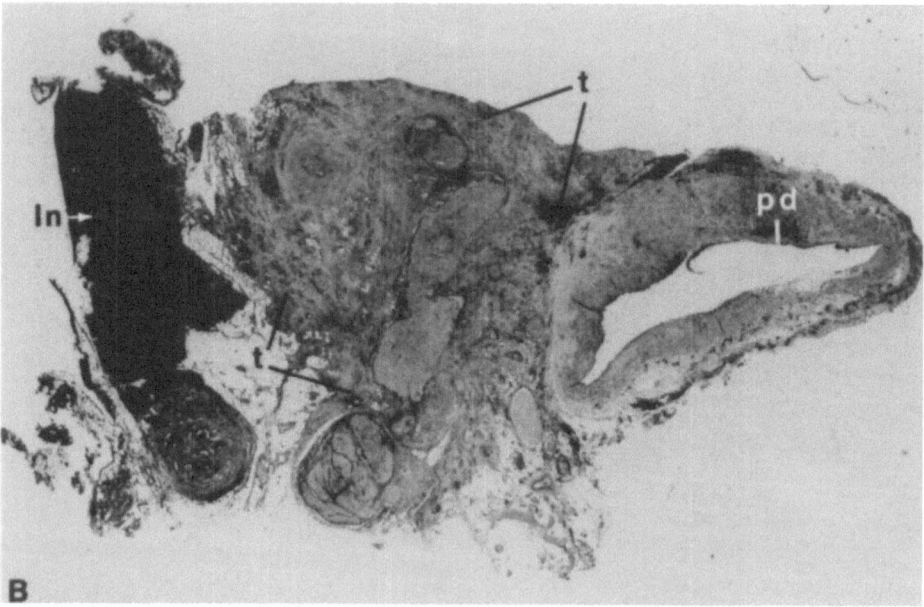

Fig. 2. A EUS picture showing pancreatic tumour *(t)* compressing pancreatic duct *(pd)* with adjacent small lymph nodes *(ln)*. A large lymph node *(arrow)* was suggestive of malignancy. **B** Corresponding histology showing tumour mass, dilatation of pancreatic duct, and adjacent malignant lymph node. The resemblence of EUS images and histology is readily seen

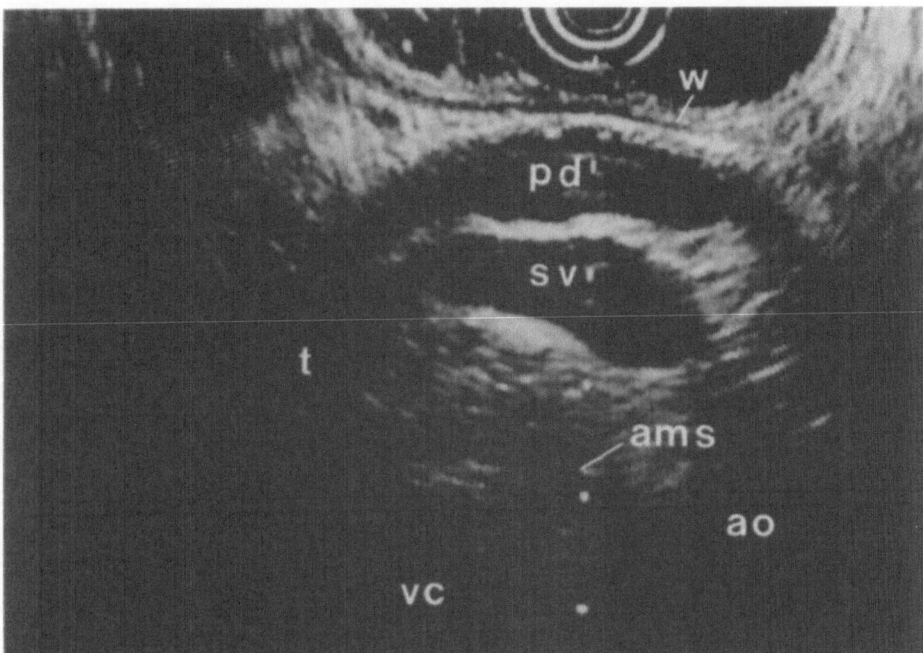

Fig. 3. EUS picture showing hypoechoic tumour mass *(t)* compressing pancreatic duct with prestenotic dilatation *(pd)* by placing the echo probe opposite the posterior wall *(w)* of the stomach. *vc,* Vena cava; *ao,* aorta; *ams,* arteria mesenterica superior

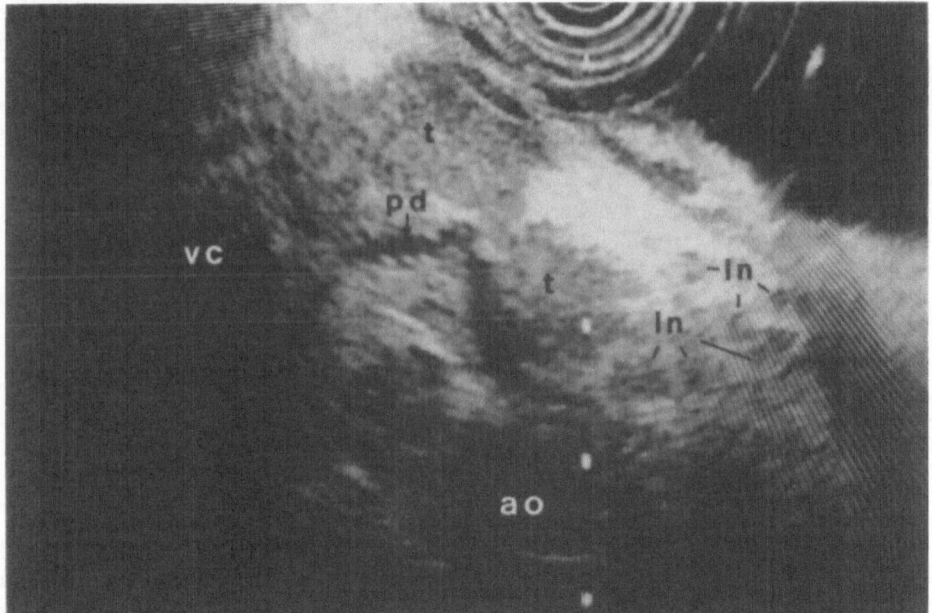

Fig. 4. EUS picture showing extensive tumour mass *(t)* with visualization of the pancreatic duct *(pd)* and side branches and infiltration adjacent to the aorta *(ao)*. *ln,* Lymph node; *vc,* vena cava

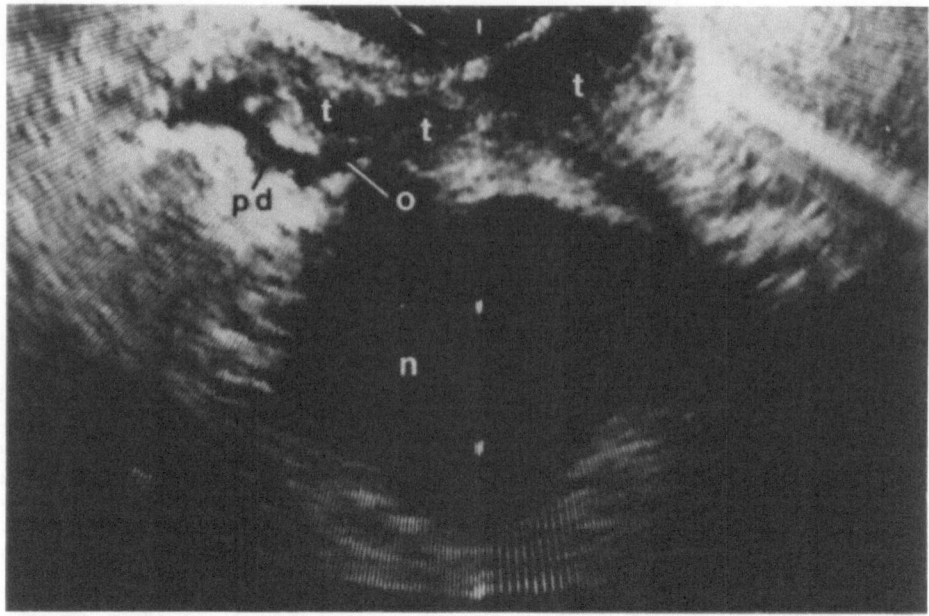

Fig. 5. EUS picture showing hypoechoic tumour mass *(t)* causing obstruction *(o)* of the pancreatic duct *(pd)* and visualization of a necrotic cavity *(n)*

necrotic cavities, and of pancreatic duct obstruction (Fig. 5). EUS failed to visualize liver metastasis in one patient because the lesion was invisible owing to the limited penetration depth of the ultrasonic beam.

Table 2 summarizes the results of EUS compared with surgical exploration in detecting and predicting local and palliative resectability and non-resectability of periampullary carcinoma.

Table 2. Comparison of EUS and surgery in assessing local and palliative resectability and non-resectability of periampullary carcinoma

n	Local resectability (EUS/surg.)	Palliative resectability (EUS/surg.)	Local non-resectability (EUS/surg.)
9	2/3	3/4	2/2

Local resectability was diagnosed with EUS before surgery in two of three patients because the lesion appeared clearly delineated and there was no evidence of lymph node involvement. The detection of a hypoechoic structure, localized in the papillary region, with extension into the common bile duct and/or the pancreatic duct, together with corresponding ductular dilation was characteristic of a papillary tumour (Fig. 6).

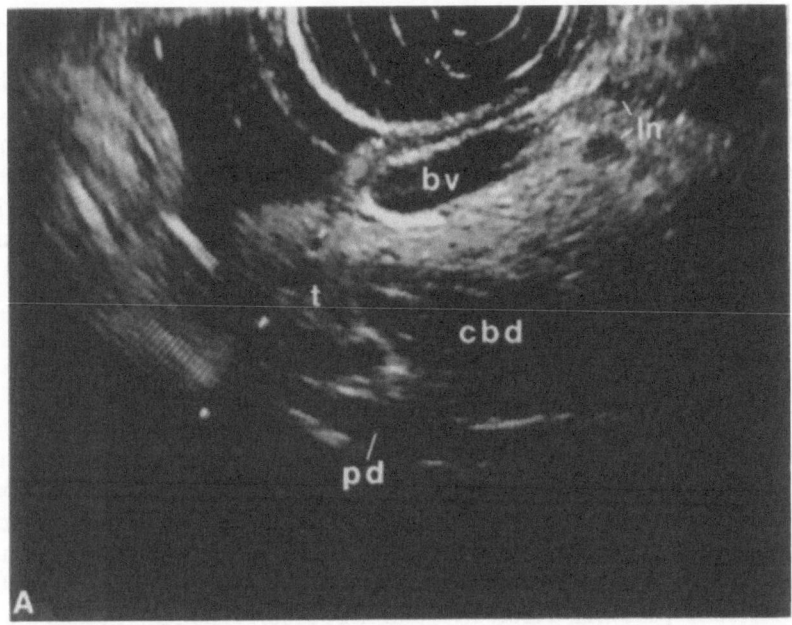

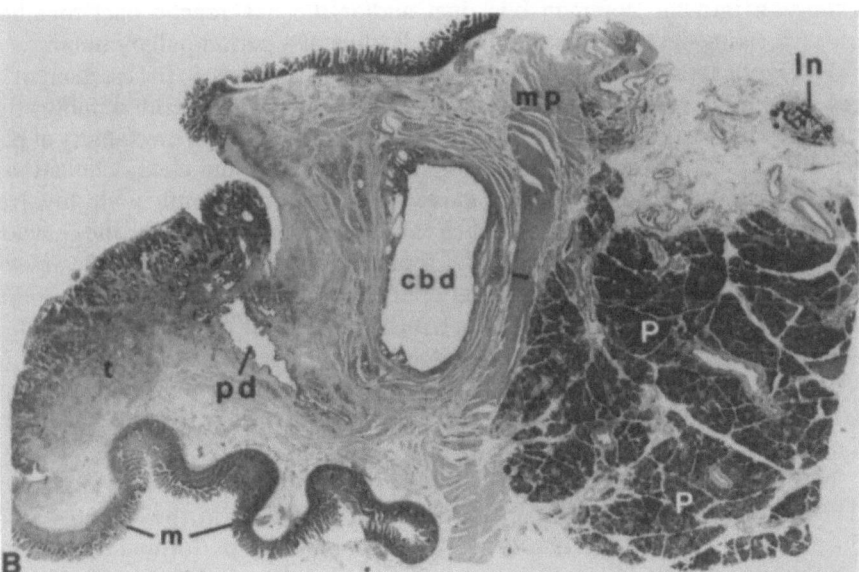

Fig. 6. A EUS picture showing tumour *(t)* with hypoechoic structure 1 cm in diameter adjacent to dilated common bile duct *(cbd)*, and normal pancreatic duct *(pd)* with visualization of small lymph nodes *(ln)* not suggestive of malignancy and blood vessel *(bv)*. **B** Corresponding histology of resection specimen showing papillary carcinoma adjacent to the pancreatic duct and common bile duct, with visualization of a benign lymph node adjacent to the pancreas *(P)*

In one patient EUS erroneously diagnosed lymph nodes along the hepatic duct as suggestive of malignancy: the lesion was confirmed as an anomaly of the hepatic artery at surgery. EUS accurately predicted the palliative character of the resectability in three of four patients because multiple lymph nodes suggestive of metastatic spread were visualized in the hepatoduodenal ligament (along the common bile duct) and/or around the aorta (coeliac trunk). In one of four patients the echoendoscope could not pass the duodenal bulb, and therefore the lesion was not clearly visualized. The locally non-resectable nature of a periampullary carcinoma was diagnosed by EUS when infiltration of the major blood vessels (portal vein and/or hepatic artery) was found, which was confirmed at surgery in two patients.

Discussion

EUS enables accurate staging of pancreatic and periampullary malignancy. The high accuracy is based on the high resolution of this real-time sonographic instrument and its ability to visualize both parenchymal and ductular lesions of the pancreas and the common bile duct. Moreover, adjacent lymph node abnormality can accurately be visualized. Mass lesions of the pancreas with round or polycyclic clearly delineated boundaries, showing a more irregular hypoechoic echo pattern than the surrounding pancreas, are highly suggestive of malignancy. Supplementary findings, such as compression of the pancreatic duct and prestenotic dilatation, are very helpful in characterizing the malignant nature of the lesion. Hypoechoic polypoid and/or intramural lesions adjacent to the periampullary region with or without intraductular extension into the common bile duct and/or the pancreactic duct together with corresponding ductular dilatation are indicative of a periampullary tumour.

EUS appears to be a highly accurate diagnostic procedure in the assessment of local resectability because it enables detailed visualization of the depth of infiltration into the surrounding tissues and/or organs. The diagnosis of local resectability of pancreatic and periampullary carcinoma is based on the sharp and clear delineation of the cancerous mass with or without evidence of regional lymph node involvement. Distant lymph node involvement, such as around the splenic artery, the coeliac trunk, or aorta, in the presence of a locally resectable tumour strongly indicates that the resection should be palliative. Local nonresectability is obvious in the presence of deep infiltration into the surrounding tissues (mesenteric artery, coeliac trunk, aorta) and/or organs (liver metastasis). Lymph node involvement is often rather easy to recognize when many enlarged, sharply delineated nodes with irregular echo pattern are visible. Rarely, vascular anomalies may manifest bizarre structures with irregular hypoechoic echo pattern, mimicking node metastasis.

In this study the non-resectability rate of pancreatic cancer (43%) was higher than that of periampullary carcinoma (22%), also described in the literature [13, 14]. Further study in a larger number of patients must be performed to ascertain the relationship between the non-resectability rate and the size of the tumor.

The insertion of the instrument into the pyloric channel and further down into the second part of the duodenum can sometimes be quite difficult and even impossible because the rigid tip is 45 mm long. Furthermore, instrumental fragility may limit standard use of EUS in assessing periampullary lesions. Technical improvements, such as reduction of the length of the rigid tip, possibility of using the biopsy channel for guided cytological puncture, and reduction of instrumental fragility, would further enhance the value of this new diagnostic modality. Finally, because of the small ultrasonic image area, it may be quite difficult for the operator to obtain accurate anatomical orientation. The operator must therefore have sufficient experience both in endoscopy and conventional ultrasonography, particularly in the field of upper intestinal pathology.

Even though our experience is still limited, we feel that EUS should be further developed as a diagnostic modality for staging malignancy in the biliopancreatic field.

References

1. Cooperman AM, Herter FP, Marboe CA (1981) Surgery 90: 707–712
2. Mossa AR (1982) Cancer 50: 2689–2698
3. Van Heerden JA (1984) World J Surg 8: 880–888
4. Gall FP, Zirngibl H, Gebhart R (eds) (1984) Chirurgie des exokrinen Pankreas. Thieme Stuttgart 235–236
5. Lutz H, Lux G, Heyder N (1983) Ultrasound Med Biol 9: 503–507
6. Di Magno, Regan PT, Clain JE (1982) Gastroenterology 83: 824
7. Lux G, Heyder N, Demling L (1982) Endoscopy 4: 220–225
8. Heyder N, Lutz H, Lux G (1983) Ultraschall 4: 85–91
9. Classen M, Strohm WD, Kurtz W (1984) Scand J Gastroenterol (suppl 94) 19: 77–84
10. Fukuda M, Nakano Y, Saito K, Hirata K, Terada S, Urushizaki I (1984) Scand J Gastroenterol (suppl 94) 19: 65–76
11. Heyder N, Lutz H, Lux G, Demling L (1984) Scand J Gastroenterol (suppl 94) 19: 85–90
12. Tio TL, Tytgat GN (1984) 4: 220–225
13. Yasuda K, Tanaka Y, Fujimoto S, Nakajima N, Kawai K (1984) Scand J Gastroenterol (suppl 102) 19: 9–17
14. Strohm WD, Kurtz W, Hagenmüller F, Classen M (1984) Scand J Gastroenterol (suppl 102) 19: 18–23

VI Endoscopic Ultrasonography of Bile Duct Malignancy and the Preoperative Assessment of Local Resectability

Conventional ultrasonography is accurate in detecting dilatation of the biliary tree and in localizing the site of proximal ductular abnormality [1–4]. Lesions of the distal common bile duct cannot be adequately visualized by conventional ultrasonography because of interfering bowel gas and/or obesity. Moreover, delineation of the extent of the primary bile duct lesion may be difficult.

Endoscopic ultrasonography (EUS) may provide accurate visualization of biliopancreatic lesions because of its ability to come in close contact with the target lesions through the gastrointestinal lumen with a high-frequency ultrasonic beam [5–10].

The aim of this study was to assess prospectively the accuracy and limitations of this new diagnostic modality, particularly in preoperatively assessing the local resectability of biliary malignancy.

Materials and Methods

Between April 1983 and October 1985, EUS was performed in 30 patients suspected of having a biliary malignancy at conventional ultrasound, computerized tomography (CT), and/or endoscopic retrograde cholangiopancreatography (ERCP). The study included 20 patients who underwent surgery.

To compare the findings of EUS in vivo (preoperative EUS) and in vitro, four fresh surgical resection specimens were examined (EUS of resection material). The results of EUS were compared with detailed histology of the resection specimens.

All studies were performed with an Olympus 3rd generation EU-M1 prototype echoendoscope or a 4th generation GF-EU-M2 echoendoscope with a 360° sector sonographic view. By placing the echoprobe opposite the small curvature of the corpus and antrum of the stomach, the hepatic ducts, particularly at the region of the bifurcation, could be visualized. For evaluation of the common bile duct, the echoendoscope had to be introduced in the duodenal bulb and/or, in the second part of the duodenum. By using the portal vein and/or splenic vein as landmarks, the common bile duct could readily be recognized. Complications were not encountered in this study.

The following criteria were used in assessing the local resectability of Klatskin tumours:

A tumour was considered locally resectable when the mass lesion was clearly and sharply delineated with or without circumscribed local penetration into the adjacent liver parenchyma and when only loco-regional lymph nodes suggestive of malignancy were detectable.

Resection was considered palliative when a locally resectable tumour was found with evidence of distant lymph node involvement, for example around the coeliac trunk or the aorta.

Local non-resectability was diagnosed when there was deep malignant invasion into the surrounding tissues, such as the major blood vessels (hepatic artery, coeliac trunk, aorta) and/or when there was metastasis to the liver.

Results

Table 1 summarizes the results of EUS, compared with surgery and histology, in assessing local and palliative resectability and non-resectability of bifurcation malignancies.

Table 1. Comparison of EUS and surgery in assessing local and palliative resectability and non-resectability of bifurcation malignancy

n	Local resectability (EUS/surg.)	Palliative resectability (EUS/surg.)	Local non-resectability (EUS/surg.)
12	3/4	5/6	2/2

In three of four patients, local resectability of a Klatskin tumour was suggested at EUS by the detection of a clearly delineated polypoid hypoechoic intraductal tumour in or adjacent to the bifurcation of the hepatic ducts, with local circumscribed infiltration into the adjacent liver parenchyma, in the absence of lymph node involvement (Fig. 1). In one of the four patients EUS showed ellipsoid hypoechoic structures along the hepatic duct which were interpreted as suggestive of malignancy but which proved to be benign by histology. In these four patients CT and angiography failed to visualize the neoplasm. CT could not visualize the lesion because the presence of an endoprosthesis was responsible for uninterpretable artefacts.

In five of six patients deep infiltration into the adjacent liver, together with the presence of multiple local and distant suspicious-looking lymph nodes, was seen, which strongly suggested a palliative resection, as was confirmed by histology (Fig. 2). In one of the five patients EUS failed to recognize distant lymph node metastases because they could not be visualized accurately.

In two patients, local non-resectability was diagnosed because of deep infiltration into the liver and/or the presence of liver metastasis.

Moreover, dilatation of the intrahepatic duct but not the extrahepatic duct by the presence of a polypoid intraductular tumour with penetration into the adjacent liver was clearly visualized. The resemblance between the EUS picture and the corresponding histology was obvious (Fig. 3).

Table 2 summarizes the results of EUS and surgery in assessing local and palliative resectability and non-resectability of common bile duct carcinomas.

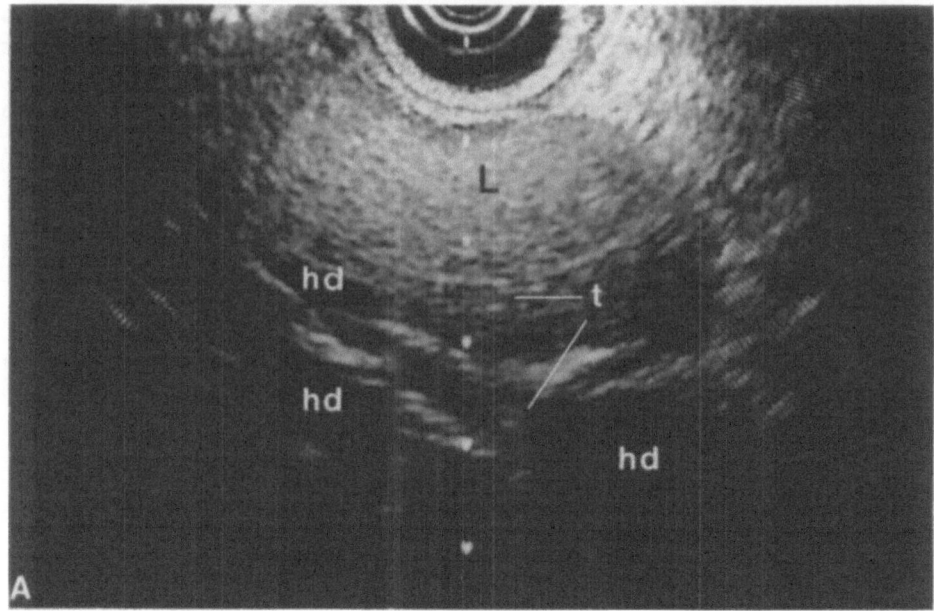

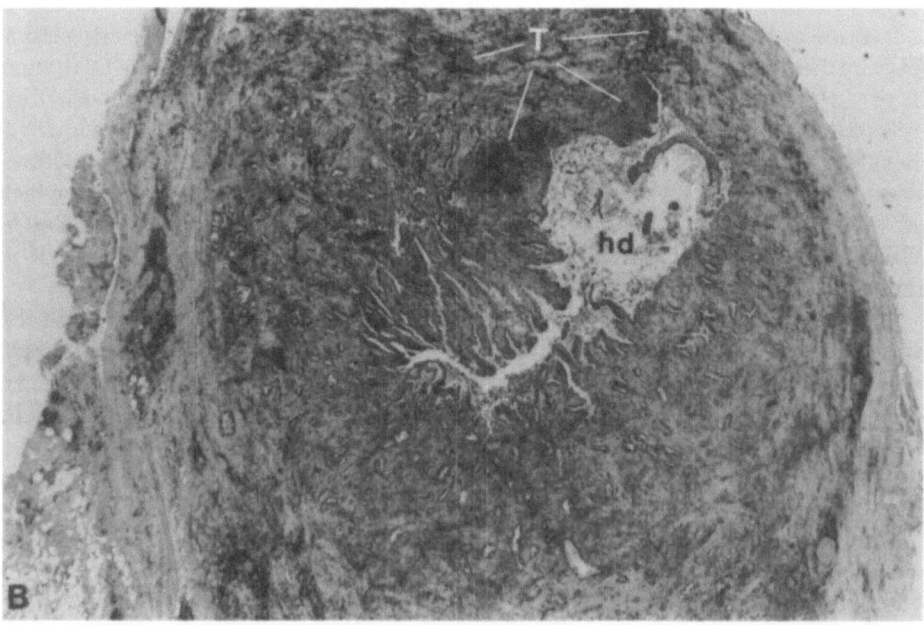

Fig. 1. A EUS picture showing intraductal hypoechoic tumour *(t)* penetrating into the adjacent liver *(L)* and dilatation of intrahepatic duct *(hd)*. **B** Corresponding histology of resection specimen showing intraductal carcinoma *(T)* penetrating into the adjacent liver

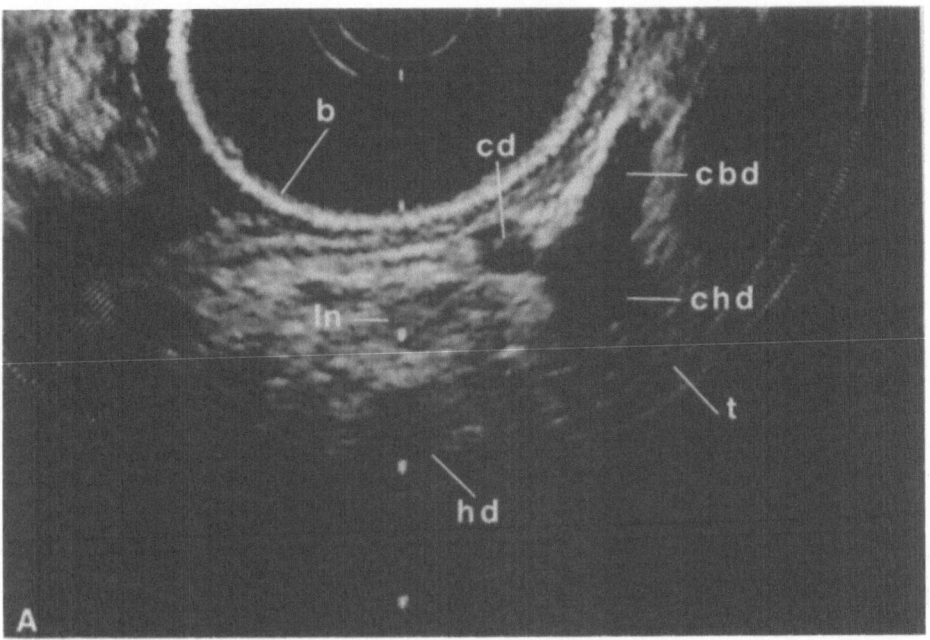

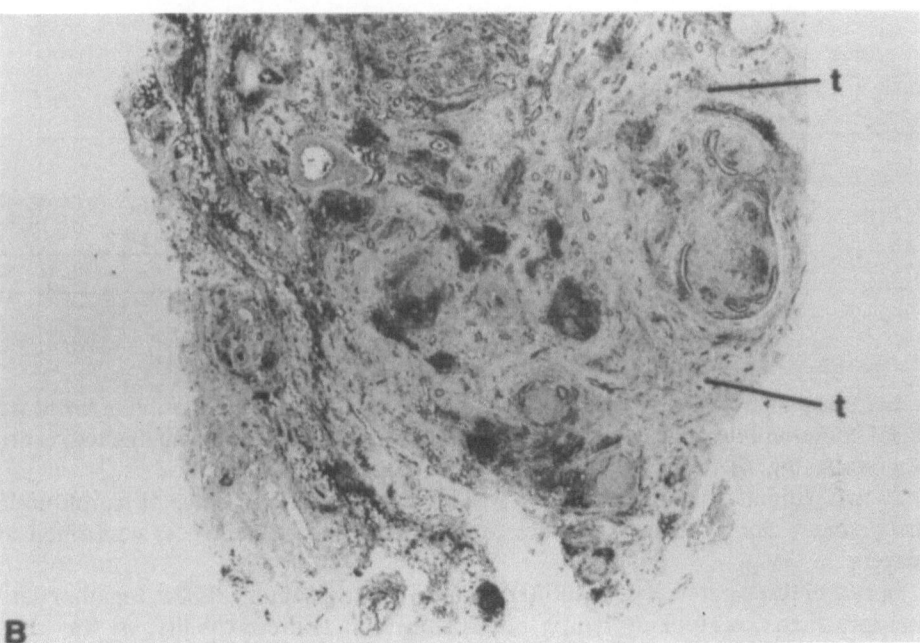

Fig. 2. A EUS picture showing polypoid intraductal tumour *(t)* in the common bile duct *(cbd)* with visualization of a lymph node *(ln)* adjacent to the cystic duct stump *(cd)* after cholecystectomy. **B** Corresponding histology of resection specimen showing the corresponding tumour mass *(t)*. **C** Histology of corresponding malignant infiltrated lymph node *(ln)*

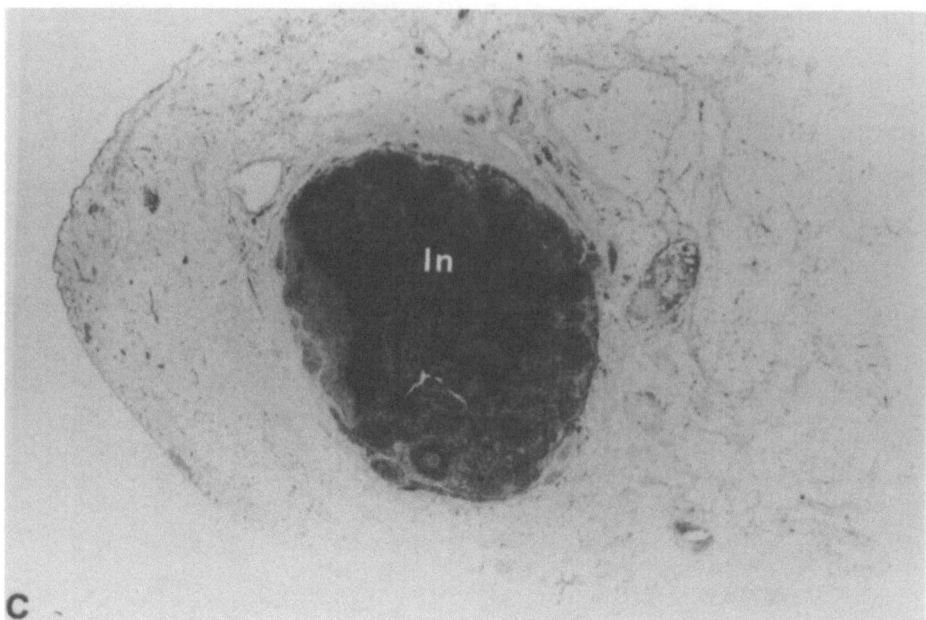

Fig. 2

Table 2. Comparison of EUS and surgery in assessing local and palliative resectability and non-resectability of common bile duct carcinomas

n	Local resectability (EUS/surg.)	Palliative resectability (EUS/surg.)	Local non-resectability (EUS/surg.)
8	3/3	2/2	2/3

In three patients EUS detected a clearly defined mass causing dilatation of the more distal common bile duct. Lymph node abnormalities indicative of malignancy were not found (Fig. 4).

In two patients palliative resection was indicated by the presence of lymph node involvement along the hepatic duct (hepatoduodenal ligament), as confirmed at surgery.

In two of three patients deep infiltration into the surrounding tissues together with multiple suspicious-looking lymph nodes suggested nonresectability, as was confirmed at surgery and histology. In one of three patients, EUS failed to visualize the tumour because the echoendoscope could not be brought close to the target lesion.

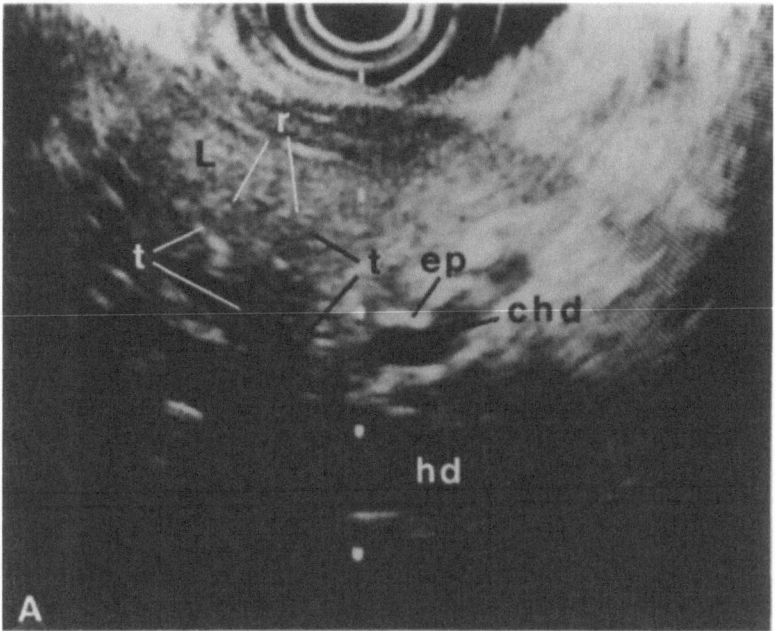

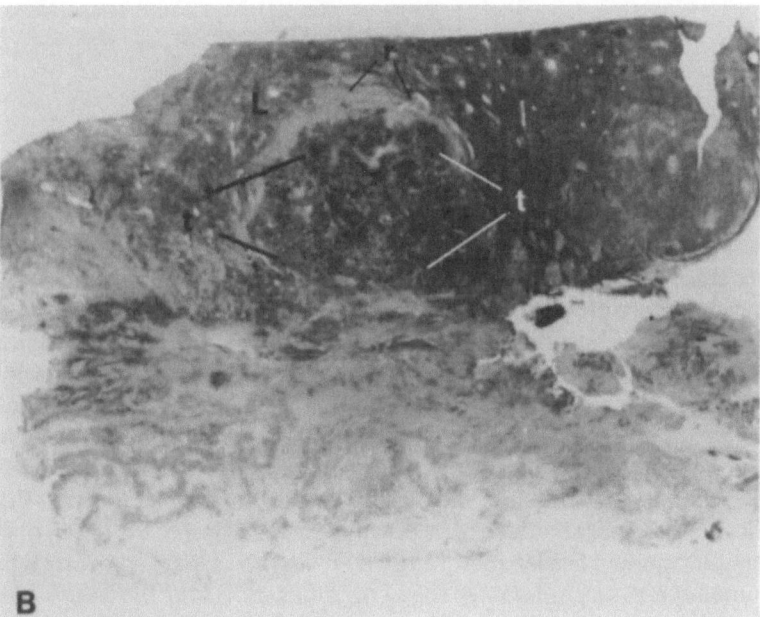

Fig. 3. A EUS picture showing intraductal round hypoechoic tumour mass *(t)* with more hypogenic rim *(r)* with visualization of dilatation of hepatic duct *(hd)* and normal common hepatic duct *(chd)* together with biliary endoprosthesis *(ep)* **B** Corresponding histology of resection specimen showing round tumour mass with a rim infiltrating the liver *(L)*. The correspondence of EUS images and histology is obvious

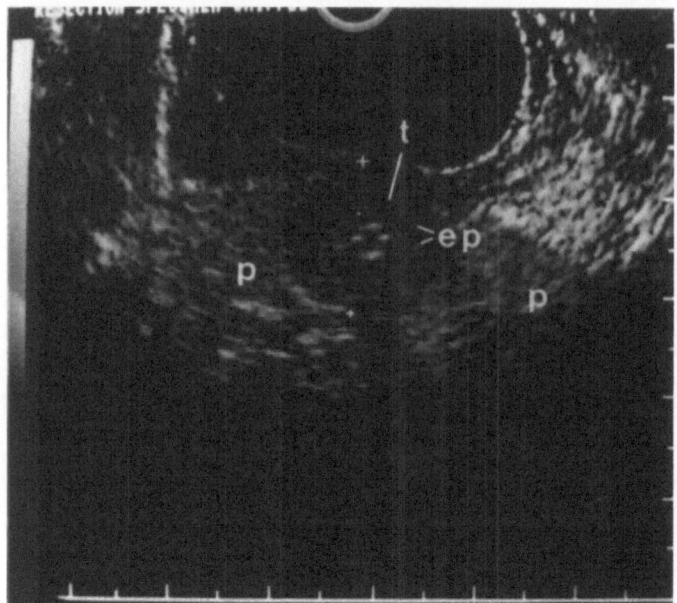

Fig. 4. EUS picture of tumour mass *(t)* measuring 1.5 cm with more hypoechoic echo pattern than the surrounding pancreas *(p)* with visualization of endoprosthesis *(ep)* as an echogenic *(white)* line

Discussion

EUS enabled accurate documentation of the extent of the tumour and its adjacent lymph node involvement, which is of paramount importance in staging bile duct malignancy. The intraductal extent of the lesion and the depth of infiltration could be accurately demonstrated. EUS appeared not only complementary to ERCP but beyond doubt provided additional information. ERCP can detect the site and shape of biliary obstruction but not the depth of infiltration nor the presence or absence of lymph node involvement. The presence of a biliary endoprosthesis does not interfere with accurate visualization of the tumour by EUS but instead is often quite helpful in detecting the main site of the primary lesion. In contrast, CT-scan analysis is often hampered by the artefacts created by the presence of an endoprosthesis.

EUS appears to be the most accurate diagnostic procedure in the assessment of local resectability because of its detailed visualisation of the depth of penetration into the surrounding tissues and/or organs. Evidence of local non-resectability of Klatskin tumours can be confidently based on infiltration into the major blood vessels (the hepatic artery, the portal vein, the aorta) and/or metastasis to both adjacent liver lobes. Local resectability can be confidently suggested when the tumour is sharply demarcated without or with loco-regional lymph node involvement. Locally resectable tumour with multiple, distant, involved nodes is highly suggestive of a palliative resection.

Interpretative difficulties may be encountered after prior cholecystectomy because tissue changes and lymph node enlargement after surgery may mimic neoplastic invasion.

A disadvantage of this new diagnostic tool is the difficulty in passing the pylorus and particularly in intubating the second part of the duodenum. This is necessary in assessing distal common bile duct abnormality. Moreover, instrumental fragility may further limit widespread use of echoendoscopy in staging distal common duct malignancy. Technical improvements, such as reduction of the length of the rigid tip and the possibility of using the biopsy channel for EUS-guided cytological puncture or biopsy, may further enhance the diagnostic value of this new imaging technique.

Although the number of patients evaluated prospectively is still limited, we are confident that EUS will ultimately prove to be of major importance in the future in staging bile duct malignancy.

References

1. Honickman SP, Mueller PR, Wittenberg J, Simeone JS, Ferrucci JT, Cronan JJ, van Sonnenberg E (1983) Radiology 147: 511–515
2. Gross BH, Harter LP, Gore RM, Callen PW, Filly RA, Shapiro HA, Goldberg HI (1983) Radiology 146: 471–474
3. Marchal G, Gelin J, van Steenbergen W, Fevery J, Vanneste A, Geboes K, Kerremans R, Ponette E, Baert AL (1984) Gastrointest Radiol 9: 329–333
4. Lux G, Heyder N, Demling L (1982) Endoscopy 4: 220–225
5. Heyder N, Lutz H, Lux G (1983) Ultraschall 5: 85–91
6. Strohm WD, Classen M (1984) Scand J Gastroenterol (suppl 94) 19: 21–33
7. Strohm WD, Kurtz W, Classen M (1984) Scand J Gastroenterol (suppl 94) 19: 60–64
8. Fukuda M, Nakano Y, Saito K, Hirata K, Terada S, Urushizaki I (1984) Scand J Gastroenterol (suppl 94) 19: 65–76
9. Tio TL, Tytgat GN (1984) Endoscopy 4: 220–225
10. Yasuda K, Tanaka Y, Fjimoto S, Nakajima M, Kawai K (1984) Scand J Gastroenterol (suppl 102) 19: 9–17

VII Endoscopic Ultrasonography of an Arteriovenous Malformation in a Gastric Polyp

Introduction

Arteriovenous malformations of the gastrointestinal tract [9, 11, 13], the intestine [4], the bowel [1, 2, 5] and the appendiceal stump [6] have been reported. To our knowledge such vascular abnormalities in a gastric polyp have not been described in the literature. Recently developed endoscopic ultrasonography allows us to visualize gastrointestinal wall structures and surrounding tissues and/or organs [3, 7, 8, 10, 12]. In addition, the wall structures and the size of blood vessels in the core of polypoid lesions can be examined in this way. The size of blood vessels which can be transected safely with adequately performed endoscopic electrosurgical technique is not known at present. We examined a large pedunculated gastric polyp containing large vessels in the pedicle visualized with EUS prior to endoscopic polypectomy. The aim of this report is to draw attention to this new method of investigation and to focus attention on the size of the vessels which can be transected safely.

Case Report

A 60-year-old male was hospitalized elsewhere in September 1984 for evaluation of ear surgery. There had been no abdominal pain, haematemesis or melaena. No abnormalities were found on clinical examination. Laboratory data showed slight microcytic hypochromic anaemia. A barium meal performed for further evaluation of anaemia revealed a large pedunculated polyp on the proximal greater curvature of the stomach. At endoscopy a polyp with a diameter of 4–5 cm with a 3 cm long stalk was found. Small foci of epithelial necrotic lesions on the head of the polyp were visualized. The patient was referred to our hospital for endoscopic polypectomy. EUS was performed prior to endoscopic polypectomy to assess the wall structures of the polyp, and in particular, the stalk and its contents. In the longitudinal section blood vessels with a diameter of 1–2 mm in the stalk were clearly seen. Moreover a number of oval echo-free structures in the stalk of the polyp in the transverse section suspicious for vascular abnormalities were documented. After consultation with the surgical department to prepare for emergency surgery, endoscopic polypectomy was performed. The polypectomy snare was placed nearly into the middle part of the stalk to achieve an adequate area for electrocoagulation. Transection was carried out slowly and with the utmost care, watching the coagulation spreading for some distance across the transection line till the stalk was completely removed. Because of profuse bleeding from the remnant of the stalk the patient underwent emergency surgery. A gastrostomy with resection of the rest of the stalk and ligation of the blood vessels were successfully performed. Postoperative complications were not encounted. Ten days after surgery the patient left the hospital. Histological examination of the polyp revealed bizarre, highly vascular structures with blood and lymph secretion. In the stalk a number of large blood vessels were found and interpreted by the pathologist as an arteriovenous malformation. Histology accurately confirmed the EUS findings as can be seen by comparing Figs. 1 and 2. Furthermore these vascular abnormalities were localized in the submucosa of the stalk and showed a connection with the blood vessels in the gastric wall (Fig. 3).

Discussion

At present, vascular malformations in the upper gastrointestinal tract and the bowel can only be detected by angiography of histological examination of the resection specimen. In this report we have demonstrated that EUS permits visualization of such vascular abnormalities in a gastric polyp prior to endoscopic polypectomy. These vascular structures can be seen as echo-free structures in the submucosa, and are readily differentiated from other non-vascular contents of a polyp. This capability of EUS is based on the real-time ultrasonography and transgastric investigation technique.

Our rationale for using endoscopic snare polypectomy is to create tissue destruction in the areas of this vascular lesion in the hope that subsequent coagulation will obliterate or compress the vessels through oedematous swelling to a sufficient degree to prevent bleeding. Bleeding complications are taken into account before the endoscopic procedure. Therefore timely emergency surgery following endoscopic polypectomy with resection of the rest of the stalk and ligation of blood vessels can stop the bleeding. At the present time it is uncertain what size of vascular structures can be transected safely with the endoscopic snare polypectomy technique. When large vascular structures are encountered in the stalk or the base of a polypoid lesion extending over 1 mm in diameter, one may either refrain from endoscopic polypectomy or proceed with polypectomy only in the presence of a standby surgeon and after full preparations for emergency surgery.

EUS should be performed prior to endoscopic polypectomy in particular in patients who have long pedunculated or large sessile polyps in the upper GI tract.

References

1. Alfidi RJ, Esselsteyn CD, Tavar R, Klein HJ (1971) Recognition and Angio-surgical Detection of Arteriovenous Malformations of the Bowel. Ann Surg 174: 573
2. Baer JD, Ryan SR (1976) Analysis of cecal vasculature in the search for vascular malformations. Am J Roentgenol 126: 394
3. Caletti G, Bolondi L, Labo G (1984) Ultrasonic Endoscopy – the gastrointestinal wall. Scand J Gastroenterol 19: 77
4. Cooperman AM, Kelly KA, Bernatz PE, Huizinga KA (1972) Arteriovenous Malformations of the Intestine. An uncommon cause of gastrointestinal bleeding. Arch Surg 104: 284

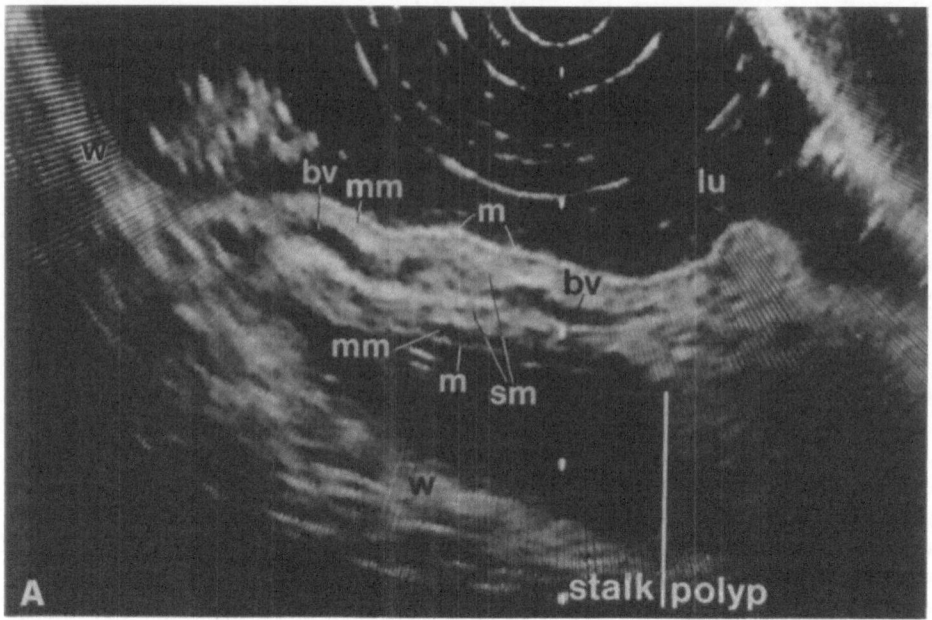

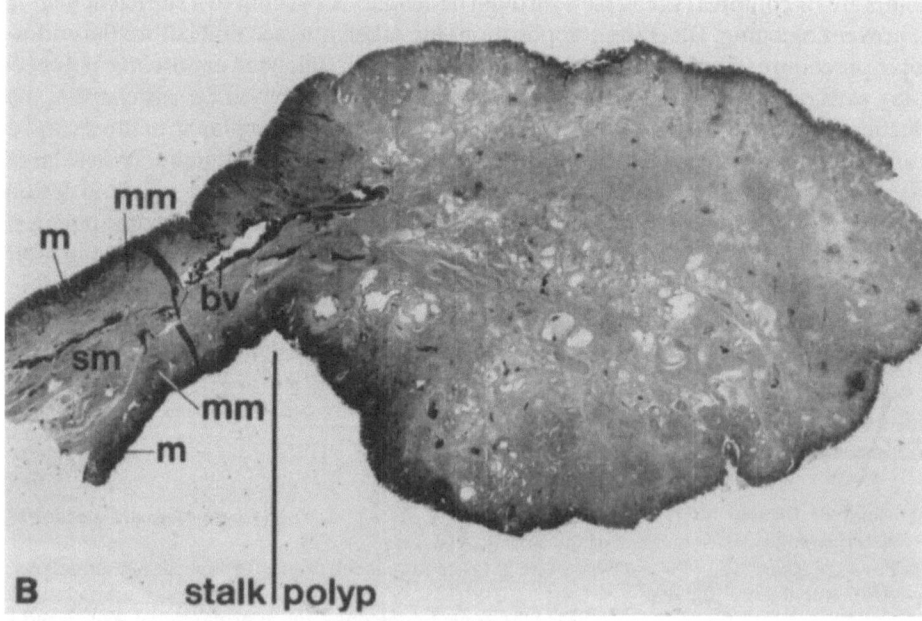

Fig. 1. A EUS photograph of the stalk of the polyp in longitudinal section showing blood vessels *(bv)* localized in the submucosa *(sm)* beneath normal mucosa *(mu)* and muscularis mucosa *(mm)*. **B** Corresponding histological findings of the transected polyp

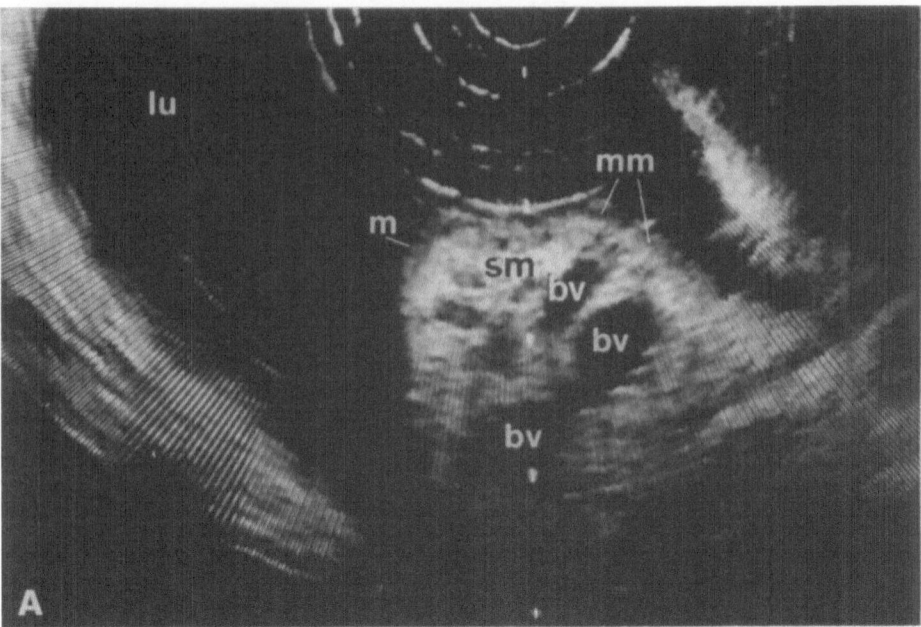

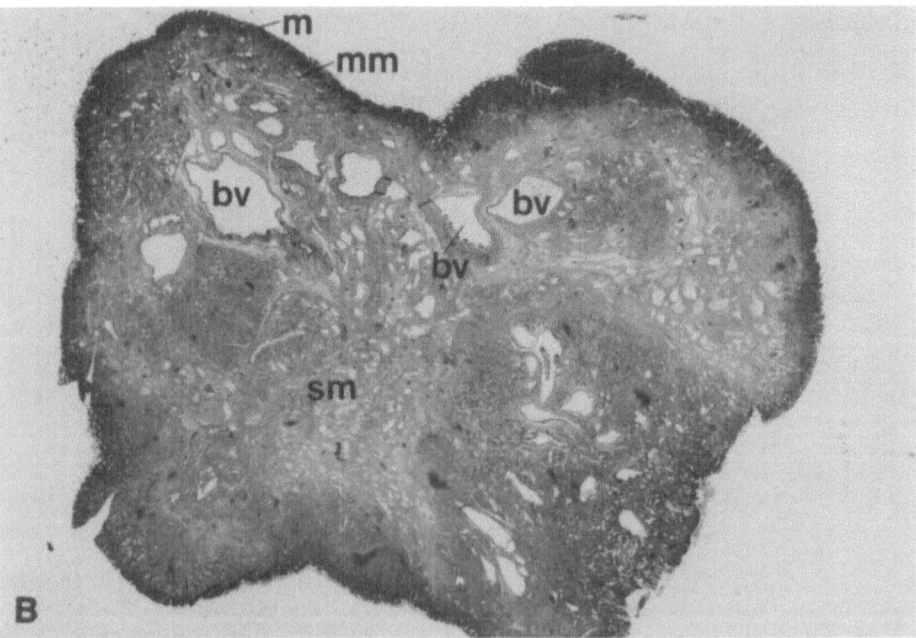

Fig. 2. **A** EUS photograph in transverse section of the head of the polyp showing 3 blood vessels *(bv)* in the submucosa *(sm)* beneath the epithelial layer *(m)* and the muscularis mucosa *(mm)*. **B** Corresponding histological findings of the polyp

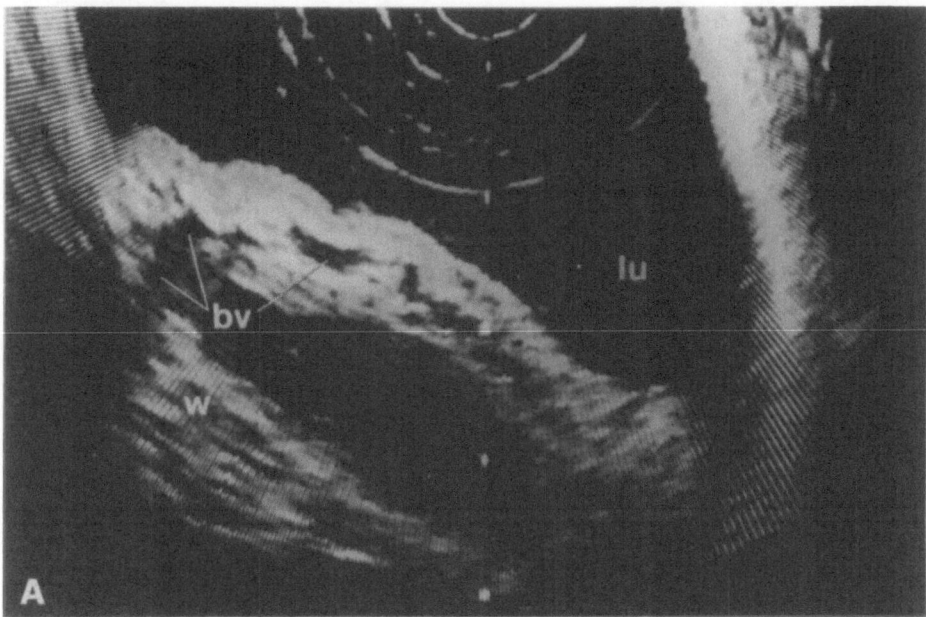

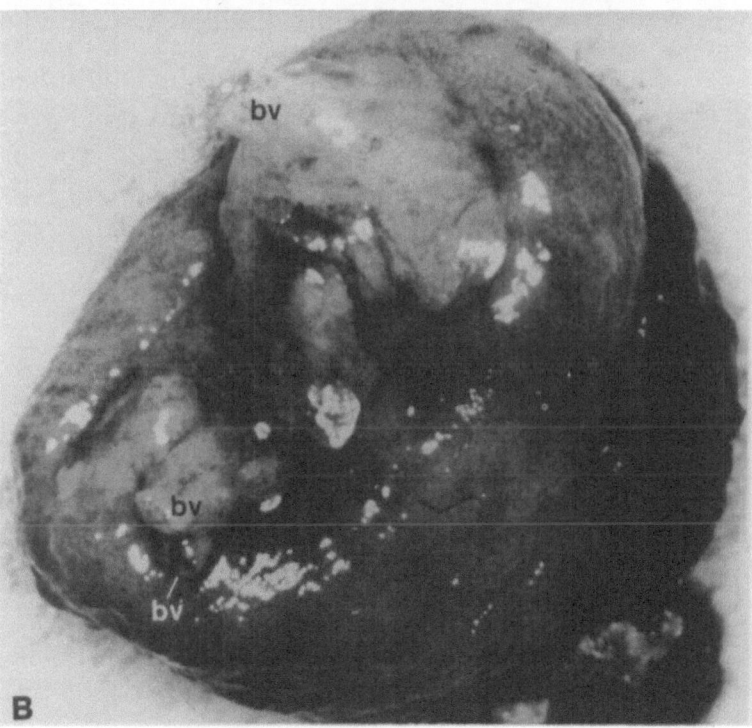

Fig. 3. A EUS photograph showing large blood vessels in the stalk *(bv)* merging with blood vessels in the wall *(w)* of the stomach. **B** Macroscopic appearance of the surgically transected rest of the pedicle with 3 visible blood vessels *(arrows)* protruding from the transected surface

5. Crichlow RW, Mosenthal WT, Spiegel PK, House RK (1975) Arteriovenous malformations of the bowel. An obscure cause of bleeding. A J Surg 129: 440
6. Foster JH, Morgan CV, Therekell JB, Yune HY (1971) Vascular malformation of the appendix stump. JAMA 215: 636
7. Heyder N, Lutz H, Lux G (1983) Ultraschalldiagnostik via Gastroskop. Ultraschall 4: 85
8. Lux G, Heyden N, Demling L (1982) Endoscopic ultrasonography – technique, orientation and diagnostic possibilities. Endoscopy 4: 220
9. Moore JD, Thompson NW, Appelman HD, Foley D (1976) Arteriovenous malformations of the gastrointestinal tract. Arch Surg 11: 381
10. Strohm WD, Classen M (1984) Endosonography mit einem Gastrofiberskop. Ultraschall 5: 84
11. Terence D, Lewis MB, Laufer I, Goodcare L (1978) Arteriovenous Malformations of the Stomach. Dig Dis Sci 23: 467
12. Tio TL, Tytgat GN (1984) Endoscopic ultrasonography in the assessment of intra- and transmural infiltration of tumours in the oesophagus, stomach and papilla of Vater and in the detection of extraoesophageal lesions. Endoscopy 4: 220
13. Wheeler MH, Smith PM, Cotton PB, Evans DMD (1979) Abnormal blood vessels in the gastric antrum. A cause of upper-gastrointestinal bleeding. Dig Dis and Sci 24: 155

VIII Endoscopic Ultrasonography of Non-Hodgkin Lymphoma of the Stomach

Endoscopy and barium meal are often inadequate for the detection and staging of non-Hodgkin lymphoma (NHL) of the stomach because of the lack of specific gross abnormalities [1–4]. Even computed tomography (CT) scan does not always correctly identify the extent of the tumor mass and adjacent lymph node involvement [5–9]. Conventional ultrasonography has a low accuracy in detecting and staging gastrointestinal (GI) malignancy [9, 10]. Moreover, the ultrasonically visible "target" sign has no definite specificity [8, 10, 11]. Endoscopic ultrasonography (EUS) has been developed to improve diagnostic accuracy by approaching the target lesion as close as possible via the lumen of the GI tract with a high frequency ultrasonic beam [12–18]. The aim of this study was to assess the accuracy and limitations of this new diagnostic procedure in detecting and staging gastric NHL.

Materials and Methods

Between April 1984 and April 1985, EUS was performed in the Academic Medical Center on 8 patients with proven or suspected NHL of the stomach. The patients fell into two groups. The first consisted of 4 patients with gastric NHL proven by initial endoscopic biopsy before EUS. The second group consisted of 4 patients with negative endoscopic biopsies but with an abnormal gross appearance at endoscopy or a long history of recurring ulcer disease suggesting a gastric malignancy. There were 5 men and 3 women; their ages ranged from 32 to 77 yr with an average of 65 yr. The interpretation of endoscopic ultrasonographic visualization of the GI wall was based on the results obtained by detailed examination of fresh autopsy specimens [12]. We also examined fresh surgical resection specimens from patients who underwent surgery for Whipple resection [5] and esophagogastric malignancy [10]. Findings of EUS in vivo (preoperative EUS) and in vitro (EUS of resection specimens) were compared with histology. A diagnosis was considered correct when abnormalities were visualized that were of sufficient magnitude to cause the investigator to strongly suspect malignancy, e. g., destruction of normal gastric wall architecture, transmural infiltration, and infiltration into surrounding tissues. The results of EUS were compared with those obtained by endoscopy, barium meal studies, CT scan, surgical exploration, or detailed histologic examination of autopsy specimens. The endoscopic ultrasonographic studies were performed with a prototype Olympus echoendoscope, third generation GF-UM1, which has been described elsewhere [12–15, 17]. The ultrasound frequency was 7.5 mHz with a penetration depth of ~ 10 cm. The axial resolution of the system was 0.2 mm and the size of the field of view was 10 × 14 cm. The echoprobe was covered with a balloon filled with deaerated (boiled) water to improve the quality of the ultrasonic image by making optimal contact with the intestinal wall. This balloon method was used particularly for investigation of the cardia and the distal part of the esophagus. Filling the gastric lumen with deaerated water facilitated the visualization of the gastric wall structures in the antrum, corpus, and fundus. Lesions that could not be adequately coated with water, e. g., the cardiac and subcardial region, were examined by filling the balloon and the GI lumen with deaerated water. Using both these methods simultaneously, air accumulation between the echoprobe and the mucosa could be avoided while the lesion was brought into the focus of the ultrasonic beam. Mucoid or bilious foamy staining of the gastric mucosa was removed endoscopically to achieve clear ultrasonic visualization of the stomach wall structures. The method and documentation of examination have been described in detail elsewhere [11–16]. Complications were not encountered.

Results

Table 1 summarizes the results of endoscopy, histology of biopsy or specimen, barium meal studies, CT scan, and EUS.

In the first 4 patients the gross appearance at endoscopy was suspect for NHL and confirmed by the biopsies. In 3 of these 4 patients EUS could accurately depict the longitudinal extent and the depth of intramural infiltration of the malignant proliferation. Moreover, the transition between normal and pathologic wall structures and infiltration beyond normal underlying mucosa was readily visualized (Fig. 1). Both mucosal involvement and transmural infiltration were clearly documented (Fig. 2).

Table 1. Comparison of several diagnostic modalities and tissues diagnosis for intramural lesion of non-Hodgkin lymphoma of the stomach

| Patient No. | Age (yr) | Sex | Endoscopy/ macroscopy | Histology | | | Barium meal | CT | EUS |
				M	In	Fu			
1	32	F	Diffuse infiltration	+	+		+	+	+
2	61	M	Polypoid ulcers	+	+		+	+	+
3	71	M	Polypoid lesion	+	+		+	−	−
4	77	M	Diffuse infiltration	+	+		+	+	+
5	77	M	Polypoid ulcers	+	ND	+	−	−	+
6	46	F	Polypoid ulcers	−	−	+	−	−	+
7	64	M	Ulcers	−	−	+	−	−	+
8	72	F	Ulcers	−	−	+	−	−	+
				5/8	4/7		4/8	3/8	7/8

CT, computed tomography; EUS, endoscopic ultrasonography; Fu, follow-up; In, initial; M, malignant aspect; ND, not done

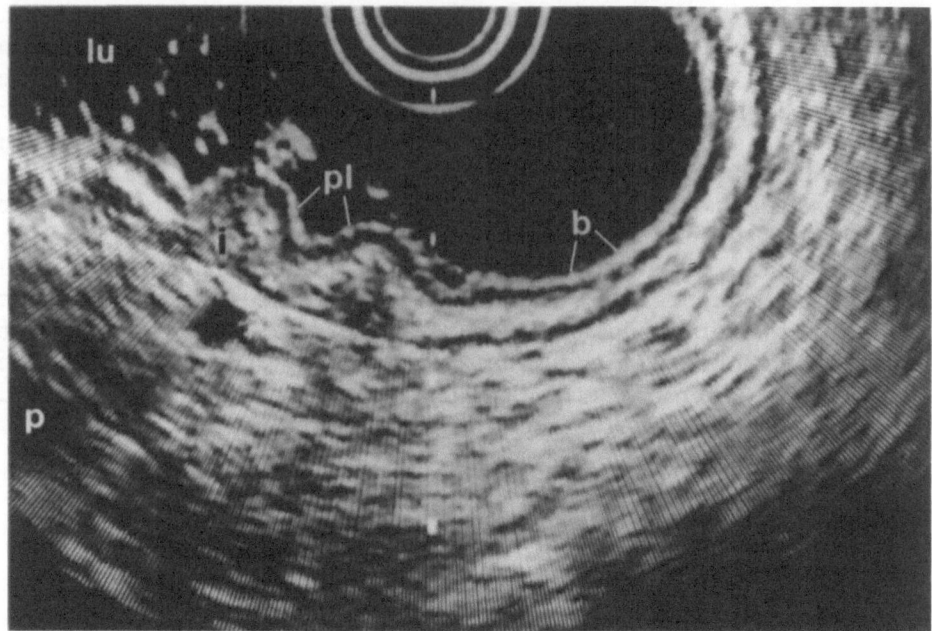

Fig. 1. Endoscopic ultrasonogram showing the transition between normal (bordering the balloon, (*b*) and pathologic polypoid (*pl*) wall structures with infiltration (*i*) toward the pancreas (*p*) in the submucosa

Table 2. Comparison of EUS and CT scan in visualization of depth of infiltration and lymph node involvement of non-Hodgkin lymphoma of the stomach with surgery and autopsy

Patient No.[a]	EUS			CT			Surgery	Autopsy
	I	E	N	I	E	N		
1[b]	+	+	+	+	−	+	No	
2	+	+	+	+	−	−	Yes	
3	−	−	−	−	−	+	Yes	
4[b]	+	−	+	+	−	−	No	
5	+	+	+	−	+	+	No	Yes
6	+	+	+	−	−	−	Yes	
7	+	−	+	−	−	+	No	Yes
8[b]	+	−	+	−	−	+	No	
	7/8	4/8	7/8	3/8	1/8	5/8		

CT, computed tomography; E, extranodal spread; EUS, endoscopic ultrasonography; I, intramural infiltration; N, lymph node. [a] Number of patients corresponds to Table 1. [b] Intramural involvement documented by initial or follow-up endoscopic biopsies.

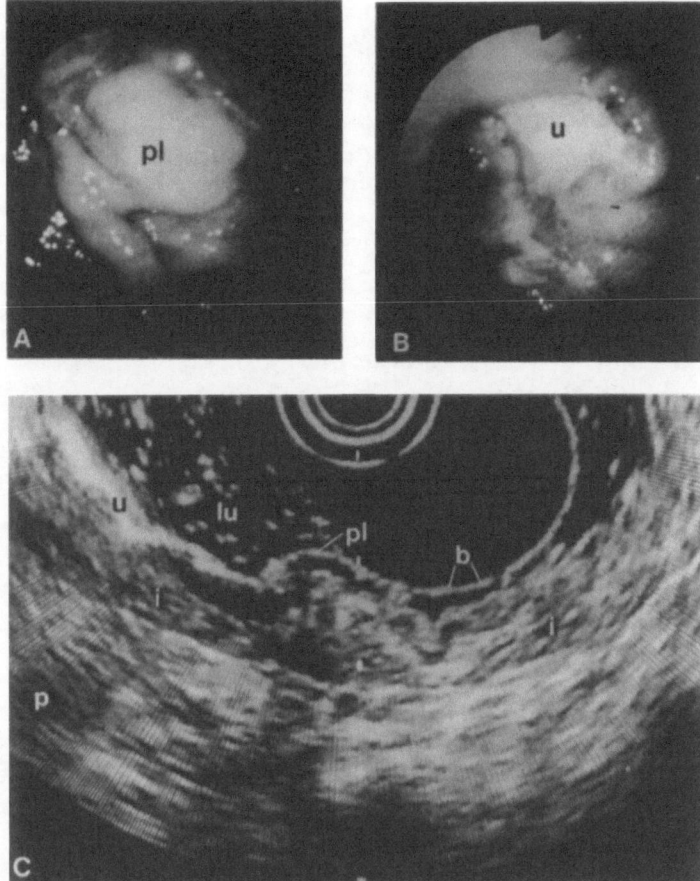

Fig. 2. A Endoscopic view of the polypoid (*pl*) lesion on the posterior wall of the middle part of the stomach. **B** Ulcer (*u*) with nodular margins. **C** Endoscopic ultrasonography photograph of polypoid (*pl*) and ulcerative (*u*) lesion with transmural infiltration (*i*) in more distal stomach bordering the pancreas (*p*). The *circular line* to the right is the balloon (*b*)

Only in patient 3 did EUS fail to accurately recognize the abnormality because the target lesion could not be brought into the focus of the beam due to inadequate filling of the stomach lumen or the balloon, or both, with deaerated water. In this patient CT failed to document the intramural abnormality also. In the second series of 4 patients EUS could clearly document the intramural infiltration, whereas barium meal studies and CT scan did not make the correct diagnosis. Only in 1 of these 4 patients was the mucosal abnormality detected at endoscopy.

Table 2 summarizes the results of EUS, CT, surgery, and autopsy. In 7 of 8 patients intramural infiltration together with perigastric lymph node abnormalities was more accurately observed by EUS than with CT scan (Fig. 3). In 1 of these 8 patients

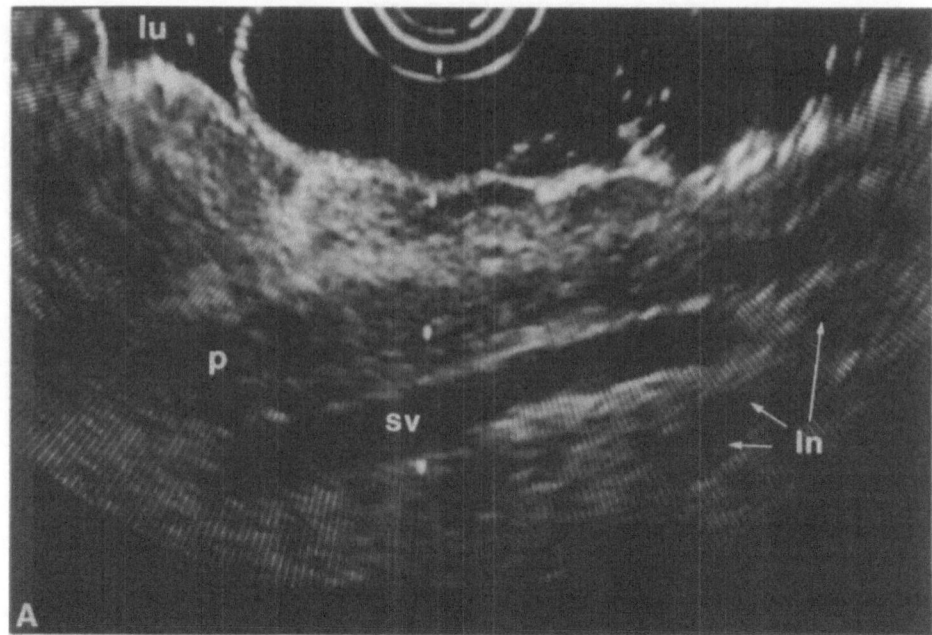

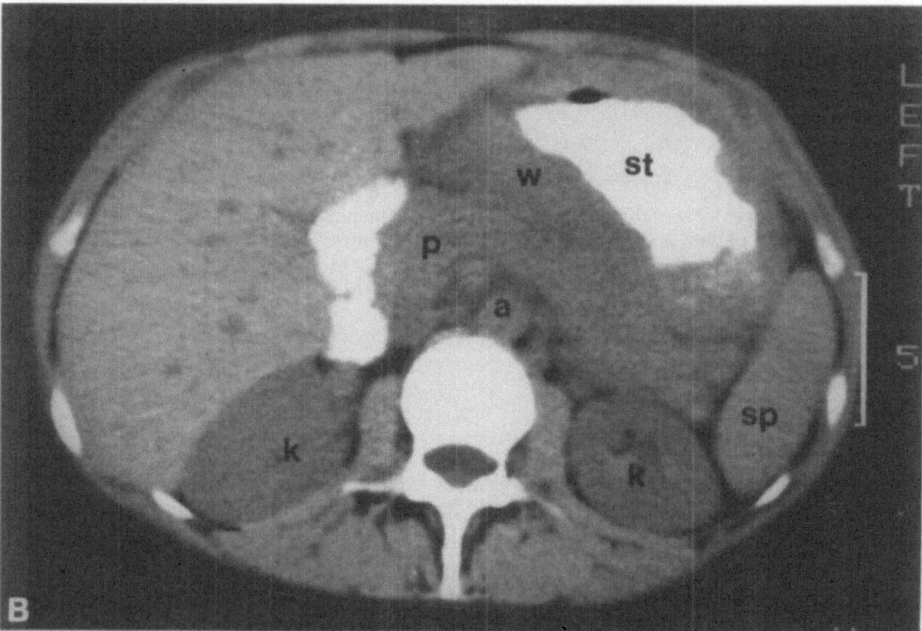

Fig. 3. A Endoscopic ultrasonogram of polypoid lesion bordering the gastric lumen (*lu*) with deep transmural infiltration into the pancreas (*p*) near the splenic vein (*sv*) with concomitant lymph node involvement (*ln*) **B** Computed tomography scan showing wall thickness (*w*) of the stomach (*st*) bordering the pancreas (*p*)without clear visualization of lymph nodes near the spleen (*sp*). *a*, Aorta; *k*, kidney; *l*, liver

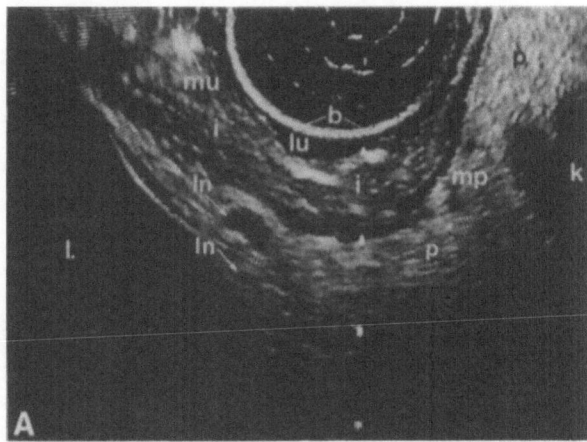

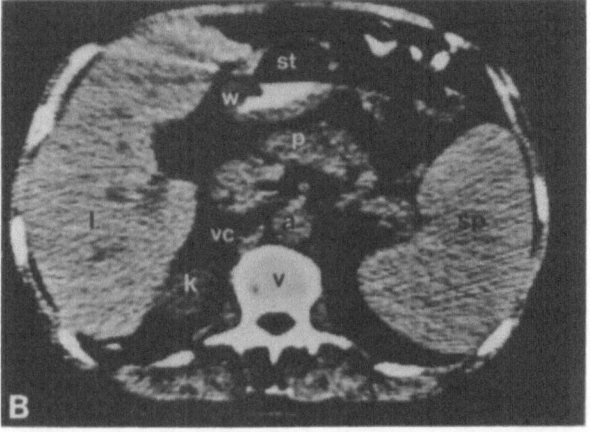

Fig. 4. A Endoscopic ultrasonogram showing infiltration (*i*) into the lesser curvature, bordering the left lobe of the liver (*l*) through the posterior gastric wall penetrating the muscularis propria (*mp*) and extending into the pancreas (*p*) with concomitant lymph node involvement (*ln*). **B** Computed tomography scan showing wall thickness (*w*) of the stomach (*st*) without visualization of infiltration into the pancreas (*p*). *a,* Aorta; *vc,* vena cava; *sp,* spleen; *l,* liver; *k,* kidney

(patient 3) EUS failed to visualize both the intramural infiltration and the lymph node involvement. In 4 of 8 patients extranodal spread was clearly visualized. Endoscopic ultrasonography findings of nonresectability, that is, infiltration into the pancreas and the lesser curvature of the stomach, or around the celiac trunk and the splenic artery, were confirmed in 2 of 3 patients at surgical exploration and in 1 patient at autopsy. In these 3 patients CT scan failed to document local inoperability (Fig. 4). In 1 patient EUS documented lymph node abnormalities smaller than 5 mm in diameter, which were confirmed by detailed histologic examination of the autopsy specimen. Lymph nodes with inhomogeneous hypoechoic echopatterns and clearly demarcated borders were considered suggestive of malignancy. Homogeneous echopatterns with more hyperechogenicity are more indicative of reactive inflammatory lymph node enlargement (Fig. 5). Computed tomography scan found intramural infiltration in 3 of 8 patients, extranodal spread in 1 patient, and lymph node enlargement in 5 of 8 patients.

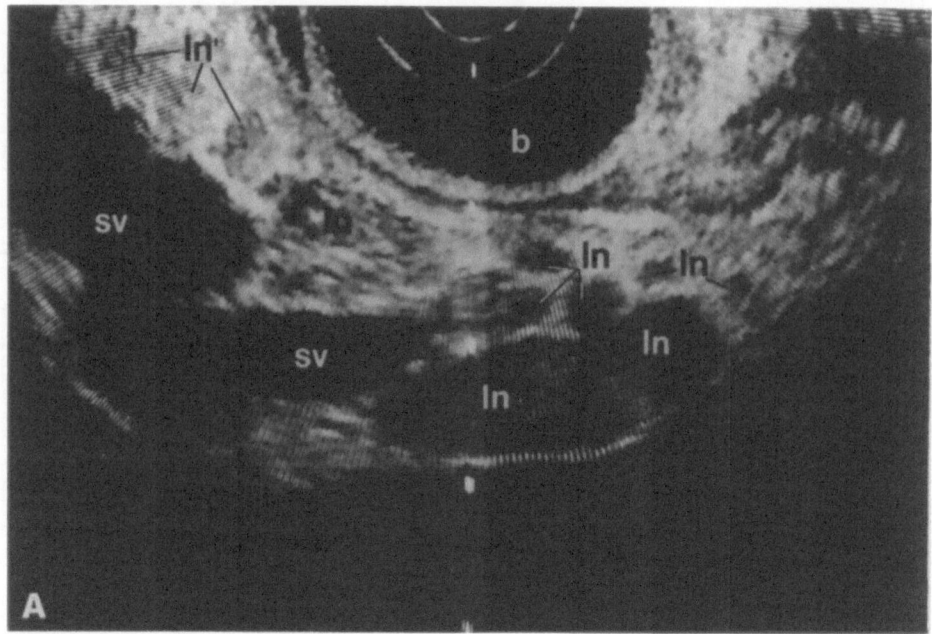

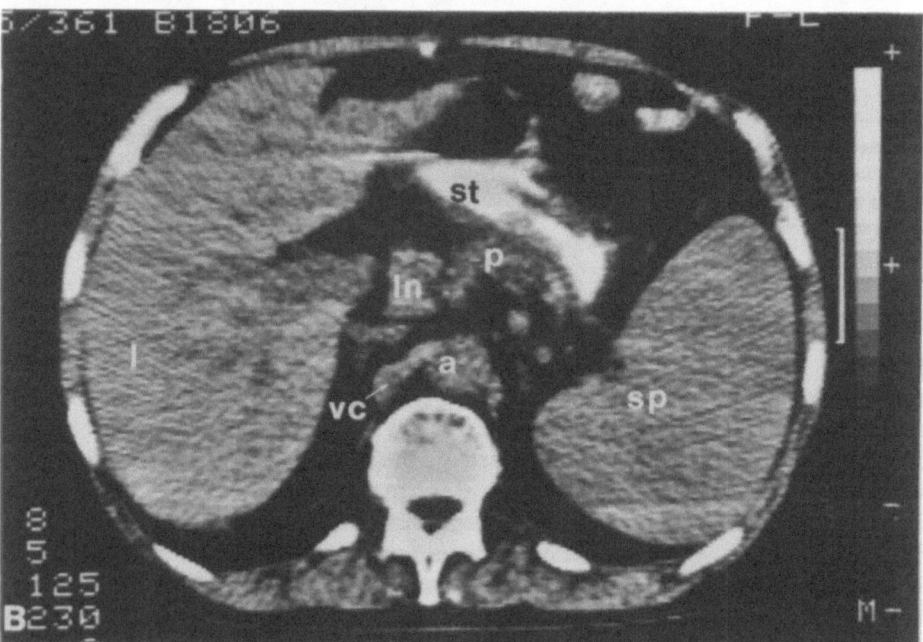

Fig. 5. A Endoscopic ultrasonogram of multiple lymph nodes (*ln*) showing inhomogeneous hypoechoic echopatterns with clearly demarcated borders near the splenic vein (*sv*) highly suspect for malignancy as opposed to contrasting lymph nodes (*ln**) with homogeneous, more hyperechoic structures indicative of benignancy. **B** Computed tomography scan showing a single enlarged para-aortic lymph node left of the aorta and discretely enlarged lymph nodes near the splenic hilum

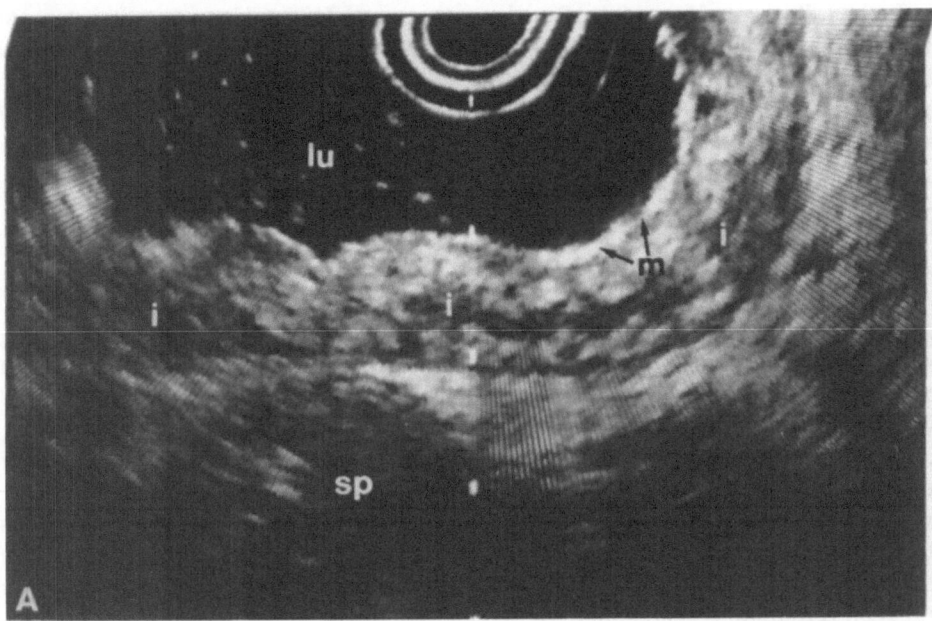

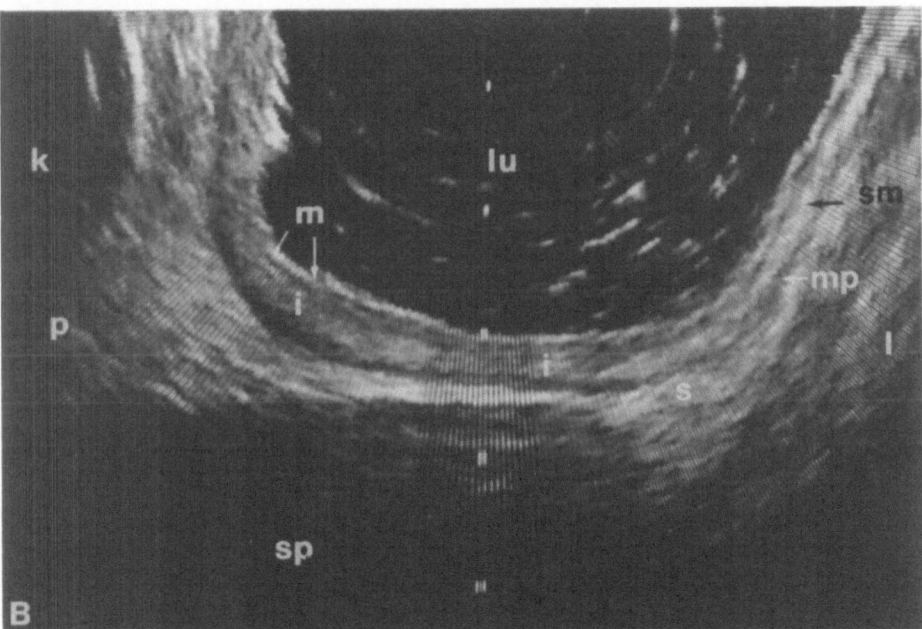

Fig. 6. A Endoscopic ultrasonogram of extensive transmural infiltration of the gastric wall (*i*) bordering the spleen (*sp*) and the left lobe of the liver (*l*) before chemotherapy. **B** Obvious reduction of infiltration after chemotherapy. *lu,* Lumen; *m,* mucosa; *mp,* muscularis propria; *s,* serosa; *sm,* submucosa

In the follow-up of 6 patients after chemotherapy, EUS could accurately document the response to therapy because of its ability to visualize the reduction of intramural infiltration (Fig. 6) and the decrease of the size of lymph nodes. In all of these 6 patients endoscopic gross appearance and biopsy specimens showed no evidence of residual malignancy because remaining intramural infiltration was buried beneath normal underlying mucosa.

Discussion

In this study we have demonstrated that EUS provides accurate detection and staging of NHL of the stomach because of its ability to clearly visualize intramural infiltration and adjacent perigastric lymph node involvement. The longitudinal extent and the depth of infiltration of such malignancy can accurately be demonstrated. Moreover, infiltration beyond normal underlying mucosa may readily be recognized. This is of utmost importance, particularly for those patients who do not have endoscopic or radiographic evidence of mucosal involvement. Endoscopic ultrasonography appears to be superior not only in detection and staging but also in follow-up, inasmuch as endoscopy and barium meal studies can only visualize mucosal abnormalities. Even CT scan is frequently inadequate for detection of intramural and extramural infiltration of malignancy and its adjacent lymph node involvement. In contrast, lymph nodes immediately adjacent to the gastric wall can clearly be visualized by EUS; in more distant nodes, however, CT scan is superior because of the limited penetration of the ultrasonic beam.

In the assessment of local resectability, EUS appears to be the most accurate diagnostic procedure because of its detailed visualization of penetration into the surrounding tissues and organs. Evidence of local nonresectability is based on infiltration into the pancreas and the lesser curvature area or around the celiac trunk and the splenic artery. Because of the high resolution of this real-time, mechanical-sector, sonographic instrument, intramural lesions or lymph node abnormalities even smaller than 5 mm in diameter can accurately be detected. This appears to be very important because even small lymph nodes can be infiltrated with malignancy. Further studies in a large number of patients with NHL or carcinoma of the gastrointestinal tract must be performed before the sensitivity and specificity of this diagnostic technique in the preoperative assessment of intramural infiltration and malignant lymph node invasion can be determined.

The side-viewing optics of the echoendoscope do not allow clear endoscopic visualization of lesions in the upper GI tract. It is therefore desirable that the operator obtain accurate endoscopic information before EUS investigation. Furthermore, because the focus of the beam is 35 mm, the distance between the probe and the lesion is necessary to achieve optimal ultrasonographic visualization. Technical improvements such as reduction of the length of the rigid tip, enlargement of the image area to 360°, and the possibility of using the biopsy channel for EUS-guided cytologic puncture or biopsy may further enhance the value of this new diagnostic modality. Finally, because of the small size of the image area and the difficulty of adequate positioning of the echoprobe on the target lesions, it may be quite difficult for the operator to interpret the ultrasonic images. Therefore the operator must have extensive experience in both endoscopy and conventional ultrasonography. In the near future EUS may become an adjunct to grastroscopy. When abnormality of the gastric wall is found, the stomach can be filled with water and the EUS probe can be placed for evaluation of mural infiltration and perigastic lymph node involvement. Endoscopic ultrasonography may even show the optimal site to obtain positive biopsy specimens.

References

1. Solidoro A, Salazar F, de la Flor J, Sanchez J (1981) Endoscopic tissue diagnosis of gastric involvement in the staging of non-Hodgkin lymphoma. Cancer 48: 1053–1057
2. Fork FTh, Haglund U, Högström H, Wechlin L (1985) Primary gastric lymphoma versus gastric cancer. Endoscopy 17: 5–7
3. Sherrick DW, Hodgson JR, Dorerty MB (1965) The roentgenologic diagnosis of primary gastric lymphoma. Radiology 84: 425–432
4. Brady LW (1980) Malignant lymphoma of the gastrointestinal tract. Radiology 137: 98
5. Kressel HY, Callen PW, Montagne JP, Korobkin M (1978) Computed tomographic evaluation of disorders affecting the alimentary tract. Radiology 129: 451–455
6. Lee KR, Levine E, Moffat RE, Bigongiari LR, Hermreck AS (1979) Computed tomographic staging of malignant gastric neoplasms. Radiology 133: 151–155
7. Parienty PA, Smolarski N, Prade CJ, Ducellier RD (1979) Computed tomography of the gastrointestinal tract: lesion recognition and pitfalls. J Comput Assist 3: 615–619
8. Köster O, Harder Th (1982) Computertomographische und sonographische Therapiekontrolle beim non-Hodgkin Lymphoma des Magens. Fortschr Röntgenstr 137: 727–729
9. Crone-Münzbrock W, Brockmann WP (1982) Computertomographische und sonographische Diagnostik und Verlaufskontrolle beim malignen Lymphom des Magens. Fortschr Röntgenstr 139: 676–680
10. Jenss H (1982) Bedeutung der Sonographie für Magen- und Darmdiagnostik. Internist 23: 541–547
11. Köhler K, Huch L, Hausamen T (1983) Zur klinischen Relevanz des „Kokardenphänomens" in der abdominellen Ultraschalldiagnostik. Z Gastroenterol 21: 61–68
12. Tio TL, Tytgat GN (1984) Endoscopic ultrasonography in the assessment of intra- and transmural infiltration of tumours in the oesophagus, stomach and papilla of Vater and in the detection of extraoesophageal lesions. Endoscopy 4: 220–225
13. Lux G, Heyder N, Demling L (1982) Endoscopic ultrasonography – technique, orientation and diagnostic possibilities. Endoscopy 4: 220–225
14. Strohm WD, Classen M (1984) Endosonographie mit einem Gastrofiberskop. Ultraschall Med 5: 84–93
15. Heyder N, Lutz H, Lux G (1983) Ultraschalldiagnostik via Gastroskop. Ultraschall Med 4: 85–91
16. Caletti G, Bolondi L, Brocchi P, et al. (1983) Staging of gastric cancer by means of endoscopic ultrasonography (abstr). Gastroenterology 84: 1366
17. Caletti G, Bolondi L, Labo G (1984) Ultrasonic endoscopy – the gastrointestinal wall. Scand J Gastroenterol 19: 77–84
18. DiMagno EP, Regan PT, Clain JE, James EM, Buxton JL (1982) Human endoscopic ultrasonography. Gastroenterology 83: 824–829

IX Comparison of Blind Transrectal Ultrasonography with Endoscopic Transrectal Ultrasonography in Assessing Rectal and Perirectal Diseases

Endoscopy and barium enema are accurate in detecting intraluminal lesions of the rectum. Computer tomography (CT) scan enables assessment of perirectal disease but is not always accurate in detecting and staging intramural rectal tumor [1–3]. Conventional ultrasonography is inadequate in detecting rectal and perirectal lesions because of interfering bowel gas and lack of accurate localization of possible abnormalities. Transrectal ultrasonography has been reported as an accurate diagnostic procedure in detecting rectal and perirectal diseases [4–6]. The purpose of this study was to compare blind transrectal ultrasonography (BUS) with endoscopic transrectal ultrasonography (EUS) to determine the accuracy and limitations of these new diagnostic modalities.

Materials and Methods

Between October 1984 and October 1985, BUS and EUS were performed in 20 patients with rectal and perirectal disease. Five patients had perirectal disease, four men and one woman with an age ranging from 24 to 79 years. Five patients had villous adenoma, two men and three women with an age ranging from 58 to 75 years. Eight patients had advanced rectal carcinoma and two had intramucosal carcinoma, four men and six women with an age ranging from 26 to 79 years. The results of these investigations were compared with findings at endoscopy, barium meal, or surgical exploration and detailed histological examination of resection specimens. To compare the endoscopic ultrasonographic findings with the corresponding histologic normal and/or pathological wall structures of the rectum, fresh surgical resection specimens of patients who underwent preoperative BUS and EUS for rectal cancer were examined with both ultrasonographic instruments. In two patients the mucosectomy specimen of villous adenomas was also investigated. The results of ultrasonographic investigation in vivo (preoperative US) were compared with corresponding in vitro images (US of resection specimen). In addition, these results were correlated with detailed histology.

The BUS studies were performed with an Aloka ASU-57 transrectal echoprobe, attached to a basic echographic Endoscan SSD-520 equipment. This transrectal instrument has a rigid shaft with a length of 15 cm and a maximal diameter of 15 mm. The echoprobe is attached in the tip of the instrument and can be covered with a balloon, which can be filled with deaerated (boiled) water to improve the ultrasonic images by making optimal contact with the rectal wall. The ultrasound frequency of this instrument is 5 MHz with a penetration depth of approximately 22 cm and an axial resolution of 1 mm. The technical characteristics of the EUS instrument have been described elsewhere. Filling the rectal lumen with deaerated water via a small tube facilitates the EUS analysis.

The BUS and EUS examinations were performed with the patient in the left lateral decubitus or the supine position, after preparation with a phosphate enema. The rectal mucosa had to be cleaned of fecal material to achieve clear visualization of the rectal wall structures.

A diagnosis was considered correct when the abnormalities detected were of sufficient magnitude to make the investigator strongly suspect a benign or malign tumor.

For photographic documentation a Polaroid or single-lens reflex camera can be used. Videorecording enables the examination to be reviewed.

Results

Table 1 summarizes the results of BUS and EUS in assessing perirectal lesions.

Table 1. Comparison of results of BUS and EUS in assessing perirectal lesions

	n	BUS	EUS
Perirectal abscess	3	3/3	2/3
Prostate cancer	1	1/1	1/1
Bladder carcinoma	1	1/1	0/1

There were three patients with perirectal abscesses, one with prostate cancer and one with bladder carcinoma. BUS accurately visualized the extent of the lesion and its anatomical relationship to the surrounding tissues and organs in all five patients on the basis of the adequate penetration depth of approximately 22 cm and the 360° sector sonographic image. EUS readily showed the extent of the rectal abscess in two of three patients (Fig. 1). The bladder carcinoma could not be visualized because of the limited penetration depth of approximately 10 cm. In contrast, prostate cancer was clearly demonstrated because of its close anatomic relationship to the rectum.

Table 2 summarizes the results of BUS and EUS, compared with the final histology of the resection specimens, in evaluating rectal adenomatous polyps.

BUS clearly showed the intraluminal extent of the lesions into the rectal wall in four of five patients. These findings correlated well with the histology of the resection

Table 2. Comparison of results of BUS and EUS, compared with final histology of the resection specimens, in evaluating rectal adenomatous polyps

n	BUS/histo.	EUS/histo.
5	4/5	5/5

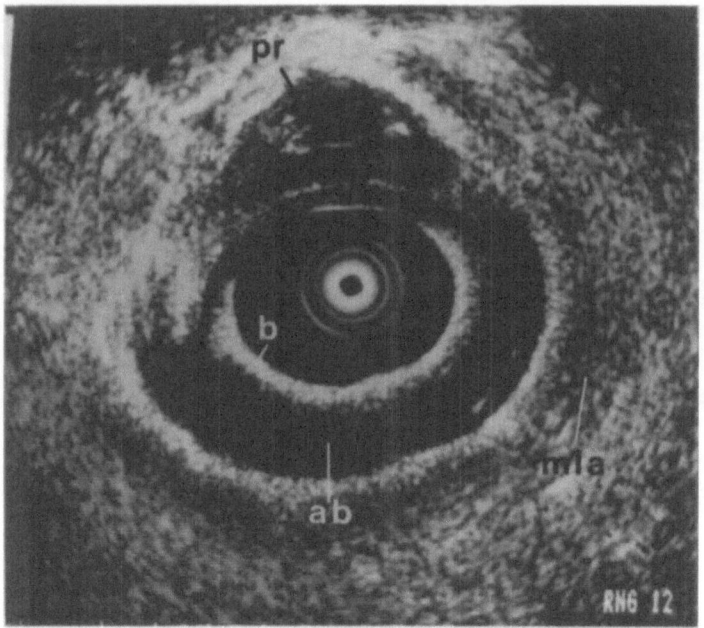

Fig. 1. BUS picture showing extensive anechoic structure *(ab)* adjacent to the water-filled balloon *(b)* and musculus levator ani *(mla). pr,* Prostate

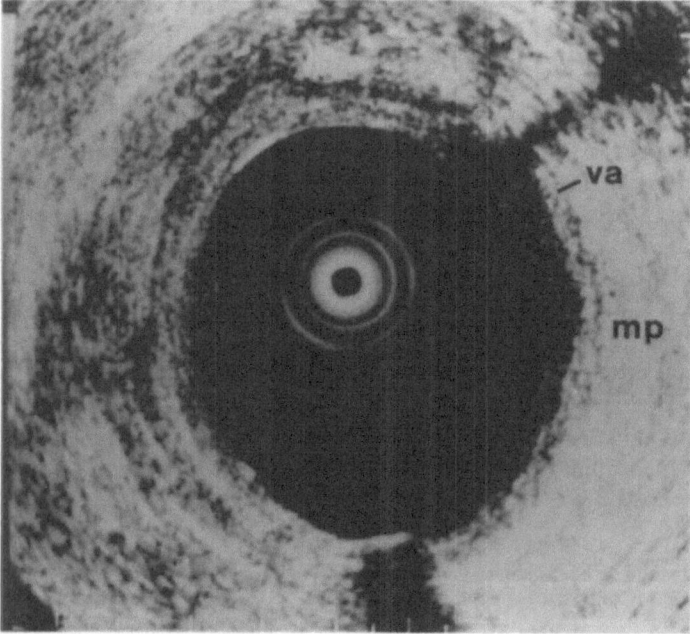

Fig. 2. BUS picture of tubulovillous adenoma *(va)* suggesting penetration into the muscularis propria *(mp)*

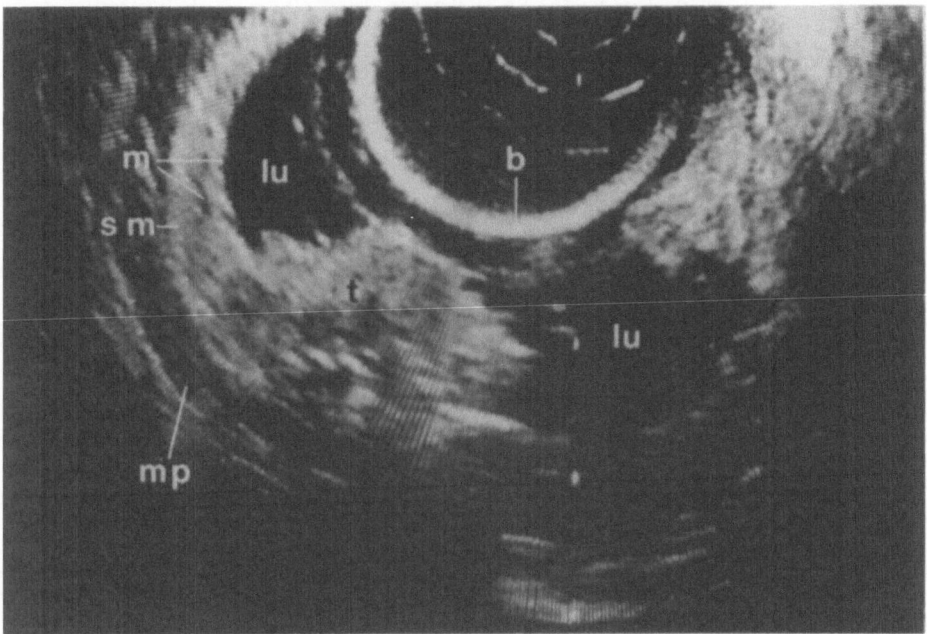

Fig. 3. Corresponding EUS, showing polypoid hypoechoic tumour *(t)* without penetration into the submucosa *(sm)* or muscularis propria *(mp)* after filling the rectal lumen *(lu)* with water

specimens. In one patient BUS incorrectly diagnosed apparent deep infiltration of the lesion, which appeared to be due to excessive compression of the adenoma into the rectal wall by the water-filled balloon (Fig. 2).

EUS clearly visualized both the intraluminal and intramural extent of the adenomatous lesions in all five patients. Moreover, the echographic structure of the stalk and of the rectal wall beyond the adenoma could also be visualized more clearly (Fig. 3). The erroneous appearance of apparent invasion of a villous adenoma into the rectal wall due to compression of the lesion by the waterfilled balloon could be prevented by adequate filling of the rectal lumen with water.

Table 3 summarizes the results of BUS and EUS compared with histology of the resection specimens in assessing rectal cancer.

BUS clearly and accurately visualized the longitudinal extent and the depth of infiltration of advanced rectal cancer in six of eight patients. This was confirmed by histology of the resection specimens (Fig. 4). In two patients BUS incorrectly interpreted apparent deep penetration into the muscle layer.

Table 3. Comparison of results of BUS and EUS, compared with histology of the resection specimens, in assessing rectal cancer

n	BUS/EUS	EUS/histo.
8	6/8	8/8

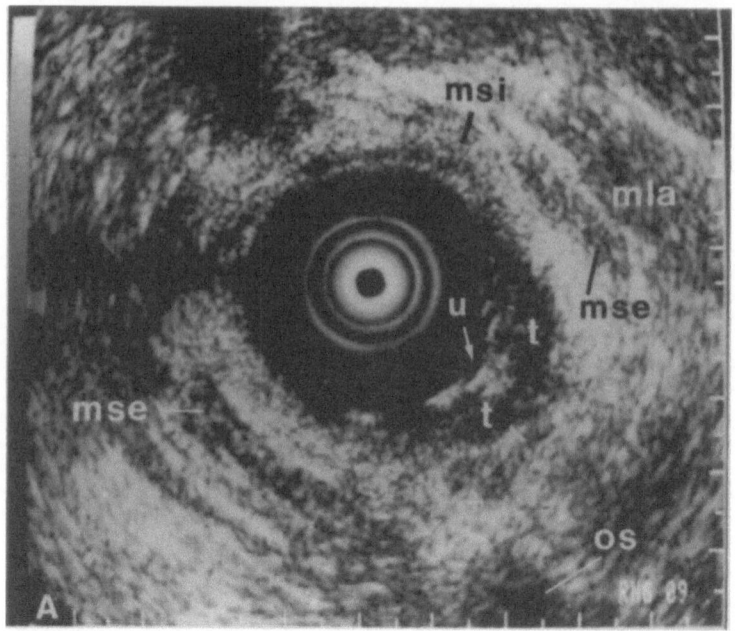

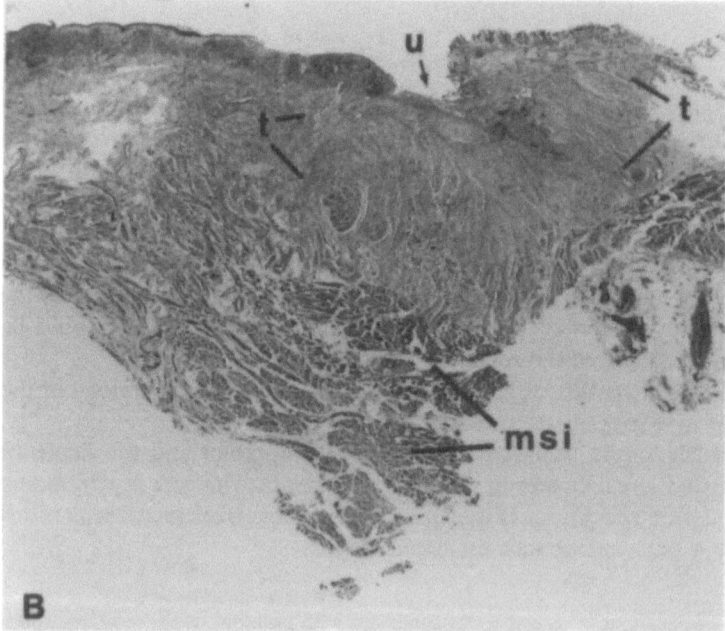

Fig. 4. A BUS of ulcerative hypoechoic anorectal tumour *(t)* with penetration into the musculus sphincter ani internus *(msi)*. *mse,* Musculus sphincter ani externus: *mla,* musculus levator ani; *os,* os sacrum. **B** Corresponding histology showing an ulcus *(u)* and tumour mass *(t)* penetrating into the musculus sphincter ani internus *(msi)*

EUS accurately showed the extent and the depth of infiltration of rectal lesions when the echo probe was placed close to the main lesion under endoscopic control in all of eight patients. In contrast, BUS failed to visualize clearly the rectosigmoid tumour because it could not be reached with BUS (Fig. 5).

BUS detected a tumour in the submucosa in one patient but failed to visualize a small carcinoma penetrating the muscularis mucosae (Fig. 6). EUS correctly diagnosed both patients, mainly because of the high resolution of this high-frequency ultrasound.

Both BUS and EUS clearly visualized the extent of the tumour mass and the depth of infiltration when fresh resection specimens were examined in vitro. The transition between normal and pathologic wall structures could be visualized more clearly with EUS than with BUS (Figs. 7, 8).

Table 4 summarizes the results of BUS and EUS compared with histology in assessing lymph node involvement in rectal cancer.

BUS detected lymph node involvement in 8 of 10 patients with rectal cancer. This diagnosis proved to be correct on histology of the resection specimens in five patients.

Table 4. Comparison of results of BUS and EUS, compared with histology, in assessing lymph node involvement in rectal cancer

n	BUS/histo.	EUS/histo.
8	5/8	7/8

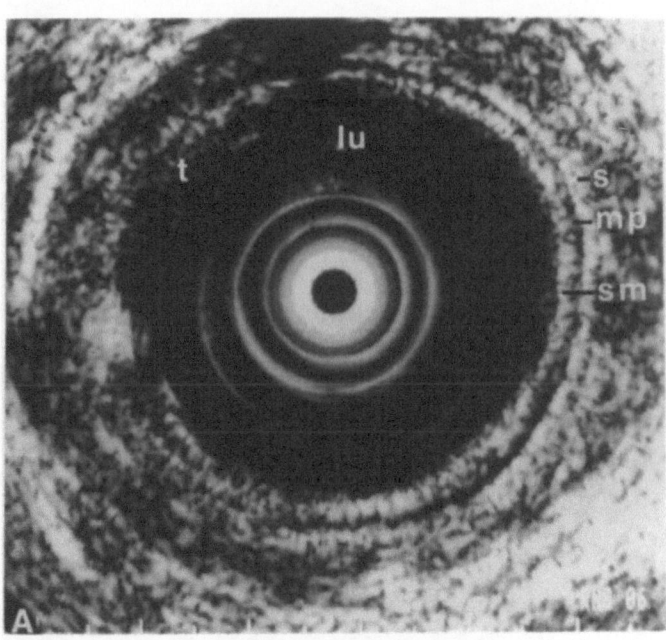

Fig. 5. A BUS showing polypoid hypoechoic structure with destruction of rectal wall architecture suggestive of tumour *(t)*. *lu,* Lumen. **B** EUS showing clearly the transition between normal rectal wall and tumour mass *(t)* penetrating into all layers of sigmoid wall. **C** Another cross-section, showing extensive tumour mass with penetration into the pericolic fat tissue *(ft)*. *re lu,* Rectal lumen; *si lu,* sigmoid lumen; *mp,* muscularis propria

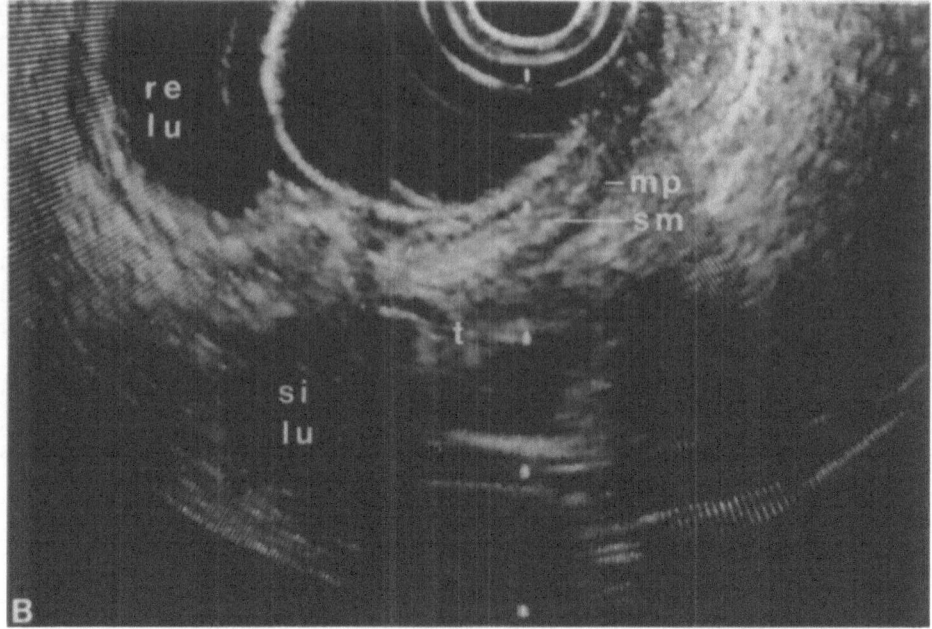

Fig. 5

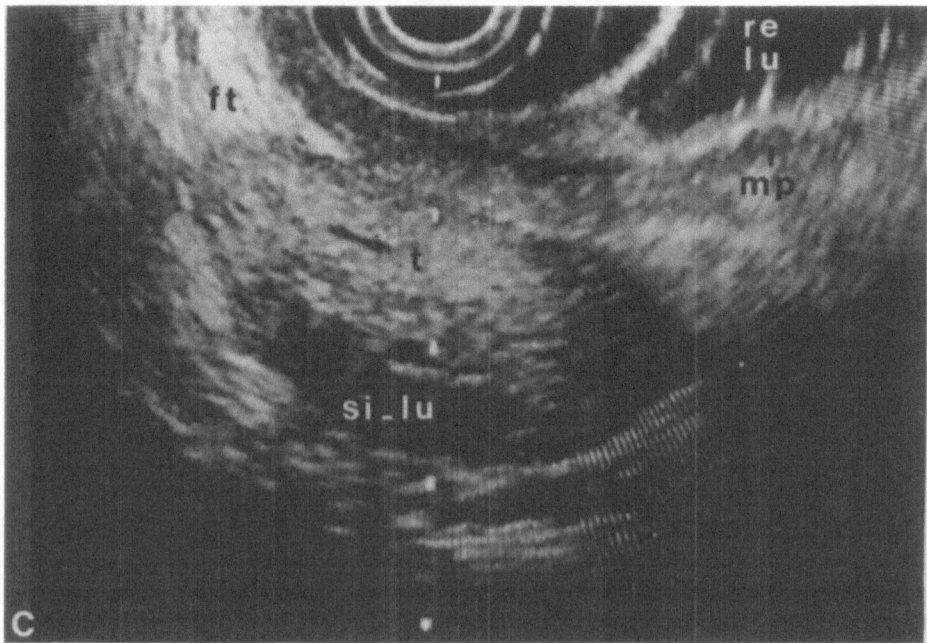

Fig. 5

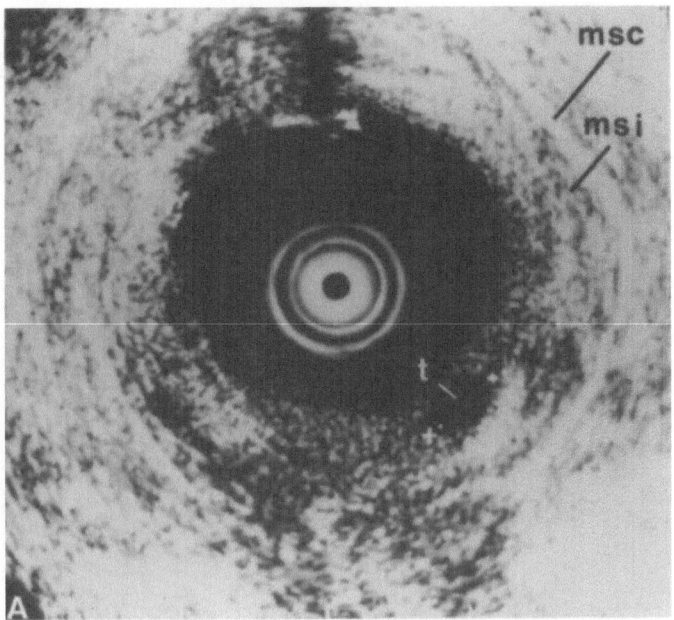

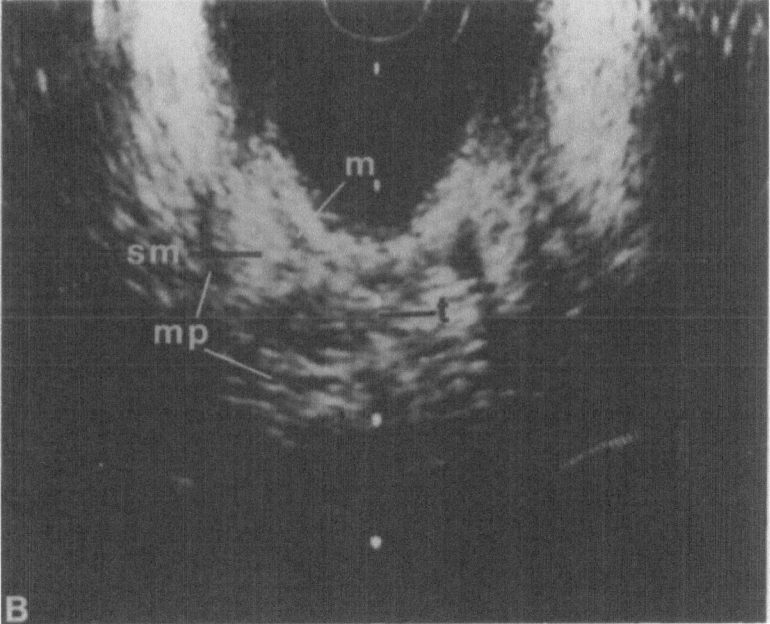

Fig. 6. A BUS picture showing ellipsoid echo-poor tumour *(t)* in anorectal region. **B** EUS picture showing clearly a small tumour localized in the submucosa *(sm)* without penetration into the muscularis propria *(mp)*. *m*, Mucosa

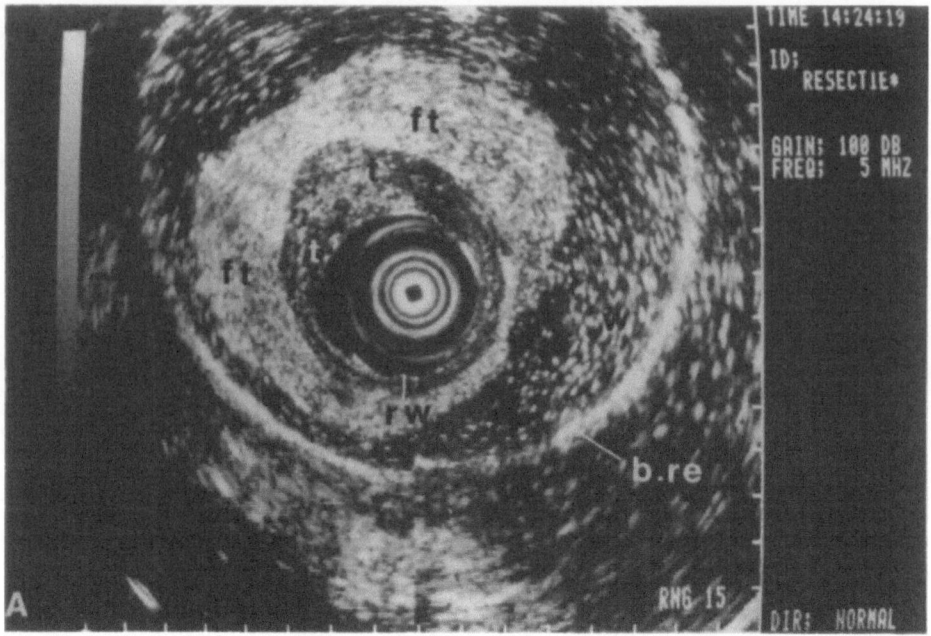

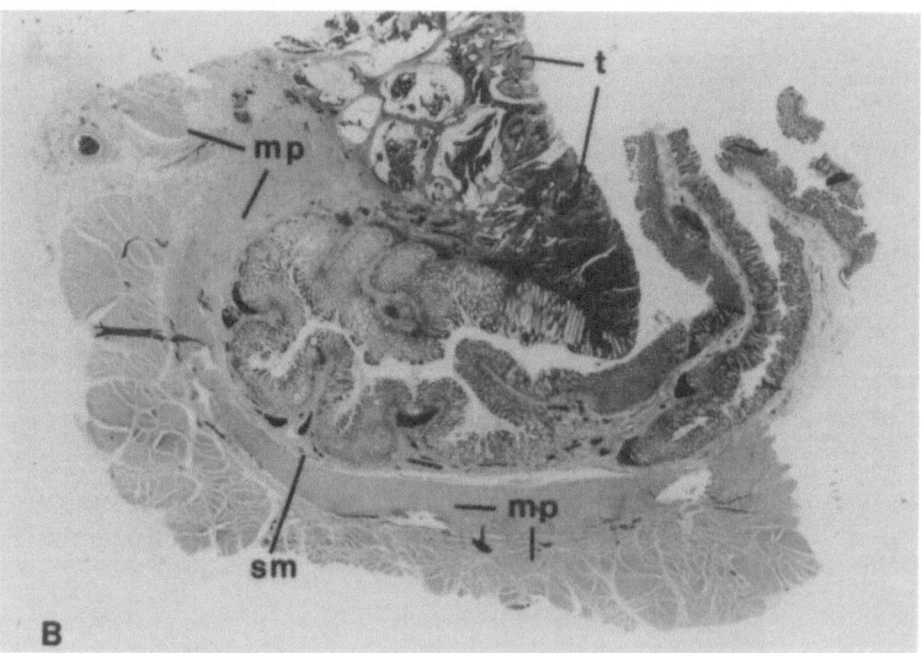

Fig. 7. A BUS of resection specimen (in vitro), showing inhomogeneous hypoechoic structure of a tumour mass penetrating into hyperechoic perirectal fat tissue *(ft)*. *b. re,* Balloon reflection in water bath; *rw,* normal rectal wall. **B** Corresponding histology of resection specimen, showing tumour mass *(t)* penetrating through the muscularis propria *(mp)*. *sm,* Submucosa

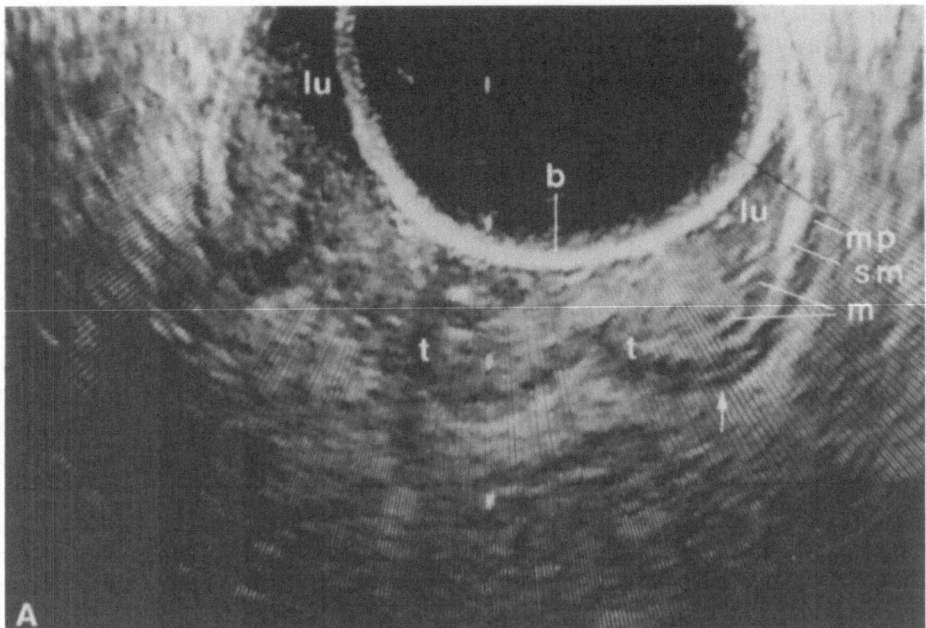

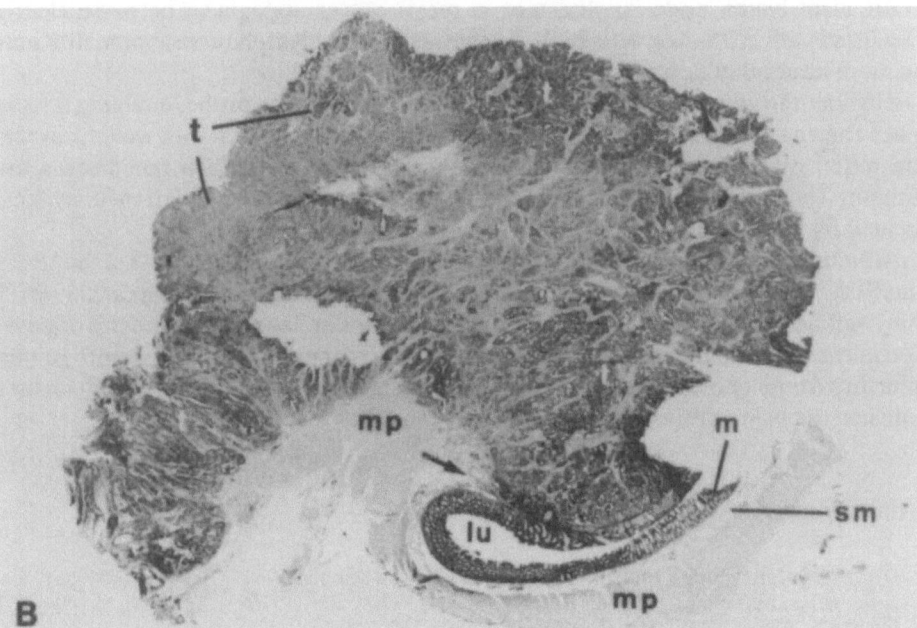

Fig. 8. A EUS showing clearly the transition (arrow) between normal rectal wall and polypoid exophytic tumour mass (t) penetrating into the muscularis propria (mp) after the balloon and rectal lumen had been filled with water. **8B** Corresponding histology, showing exophytic tumour mass infiltrating the muscularis propria and the clear transition between normal wall and tumour mass (arrow).

In three patients BUS incorrectly diagnosed metastatic lymph node involvement, the nodes being smaller than 5 mm. In contrast, EUS correctly visualized lymph node metastasis in seven of eight patients on the basis of the clear visualization of the echo pattern of lymph nodes even when they were smaller than 5 mm. In contrast, distant lymph node involvement was more clearly visualized with BUS than with EUS on the basis of the depth of ultrasound penetration of BUS.

Discussion

BUS and EUS may provide a clear visualization of the rectal and perirectal structures. This is based on the capability of approaching the lesions with high-frequency ultrasound via the rectal lumen. In assessing perirectal abnormalities, BUS appears to be a more accurate diagnostic procedure than EUS because of the deeper penetration depth of approximately 22 cm. In addition, reliable interpretation of the anatomical orientation of the lesion may more easily be obtained with BUS than with EUS, because the third-generation EUS has only a sector sonography field of 180°.

In assessing intramural lesions both BUS techniques have advantages and limitations in accurate staging of advanced rectal cancer but appeared to be less accurate in detecting lesions localized within the mucosa and/or submucosa. In contrast, EUS enables clear visualization of "early" rectal cancer because of the capability of accurate delineation of the rectal wall structures.

Adjacent lymph node involvement in rectal cancer appears to be more clearly visualized with EUS than with BUS. In contrast, distant lymph node abnomality may be more accurately detected with BUS.

EUS has the advantage of endoscopic guidance of the echo probe, enabling it to be placed accurately against the lesion. In addition, filling the lumen with water presents the pitfall of apparent "pseudoinvasion" when the BUS balloon compresses the tumour. Technically, endoscopic vision presents erroneous interpretation of artifacts created by the presence of a faecal material.

Although the number of patients evaluated at present is limited, we feel that BUS and EUS will prove to be accurate diagnostic procedures in staging rectal cancer. BUS may well become the most important diagnostic tool in detecting perirectal disease. Technical improvements such as the possibility of performing ultrasonic guided puncture for diagnostic or even therapeutic (abscess drainage) purposes may further enhance the value of these new imaging techniques.

References

1. Dixon AK, Kelsey Frey I, Morson BC, Nicholls RJ, York Mason A (1981) Br J Radiol 54: 655–659
2. Nicholls RJ, Mason AY, Morson BC, Dixon AK, Kelsey Frey I (1982) Br J Surg 62: 404–409
3. Grabbe E, Lierse W, Winkler R (1983) Radiology 149: 241–246
4. Påhlman L, Adalsteinsson B, Glimeticis B, Lindgren PG, Scheibenpflug L (1984) Acta Radiol [Diagn] (Stockh) 25: 489–494
5. Hildebrandt U, Feifel G (1985) Dis Colon Rectum 28: 42–46
6. Rifkin M, Marks G (1985) Radiology 157: 499–500

X Evaluation of Resectability of Gastrointestinal Tumors

Introduction

Endoscopic ultrasonography (EUS) allows clear visualization of gastrointestinal tumors, by directly approaching target lesions via the lumen with a high-frequency ultrasonic beam. This technique allows detailed analysis of all layers of the gastrointestinal wall architecture, presently a shortcoming of conventional diagnostic techniques [1–12]. In addition, real-time dynamic properties allow detailed visualization of tumor penetration including extension into surrounding lymph nodes and major vascular structures. Assessment of resectability is thereby improved. Biliary and pancreatic tumors can also be studied through the stomach and duodenal wall. The purpose of this chapter is to describe the accuracy, limitations, and clinical usefulness of EUS in determining the resectability of gastrointestinal malignancy.

Esophageal Tumors

Benign Tumors

Leiomyoma, the most common benign esophageal tumor, is usually seen as a bulging mass covered with smooth mucosa, occasionally with a central ulcer, when viewed endoscopically or radiographically. Endoscopic biopsy is rarely helpful in ascertaining the diagnosis or in completely ruling out malignancy. Generally the submucosal lesion cannot be reached with a standard biopsy forceps except when special techniques are used. With EUS, a leiomyoma appears as a sharply demarcated lesion with a homogeneous echostructure and echopattern under normal-appearing mucosa. Local thickening of the muscularis propria may also be seen. Leiomyomas compress but do not infiltrate into surrounding tissues. A submucosal tumor mass with an inhomogeneous echopattern and less demarcated or bizarrely defined borders is strongly indicative of a leiomyoblastoma or leimyosarcoma. These occasionally contain a central ulcer. Differentiation between a benign and malignant lesion can occasionally be difficult. The presence of suspicious lymph nodes may be helpful in distinguishing the malignant character of the lesion.

Malignant Tumors

"Early" esophageal carcinoma is visualized as a hypoechoic lesion localized in the mucosa and/or submucosa without penetration into the muscularis propria. There is no evidence of adjacent lymph node involvement. In some cases, a benign inflammatory reaction secondary to ulcerative changes of an "early" cancerous lesion may simulate a more deeply infiltrating cancer.

In cases of more advanced cancer, a sonographic assessment of local curative resectability is made when a well demarcated hypoechoic tumorous lesion is found, without spread through the organ boundaries or to adjacent lymph nodes. Some surgeons claim that regional lymph node involvement does not rule out curative resection. We feel that chances for cure are remote if regional lymph node involvement is found (Fig. 1). Resectability is considered to be palliative in nature when not only regional but also distant lymph node involvement is found in the presence of a locally resectable tumor. Some surgeons feel that only distant lymph node metastasis, e. g., around the celiac trunc, splenic hilum, and/or along the omentum, indicates nonresectability. Evidence of unquestionable nonresectability is diagnosed when there is deep penetration of malignancy into the surrounding tissues, e. g., major blood vessels, diaphragm, vertebrae, or adjacent organs such as the pericardium, tracheobronchial tree, and liver. In such circumstances, the entire tumor cannot be removed from the surrounding tissues or organ [8, 9]. Data collected in a prospective study and summarized in Table 1 support this definition of curative resectability, palliative resectability, and nonresectability.

In cases of extensive deep penetration into or through the adjacent tracheobronchial tree, differentiation between an esophageal and a bronchial or tracheal carcinoma can be very difficult (Fig. 2). Bronchoscopy is helpful in ascertaining the diagnosis. In a prospective study EUS was found to be superior to CT in determining resectability of esophageal malignancies. The ability to achieve cross and longitudinal sections of the tumor and to visualize the periintestinal lymph nodes even when the diameter was less than 5 mm was better than CT scanning (Fig. 3). Moreover, real-time dynamic ultrasonography is superior to the static radiographic device in the assessment of tumor penetration around or into the adjacent blood vessels (Fig. 4). Data in Table 2 support the superiority of EUS over CT scanning in assessing the resectability of esophageal carcinoma.

Table 1. Summary of the results of EUS in assessing resectability of esophageal carcinoma

	EUS correct diagnosis	Surgery/histology
Curative resectability	15	18
Palliative resectability	22	26
Nonresectability	10	11

Table 2. Summary of the results of EUS and CT scanning in assessing resectability of esophageal carcinoma

	EUS	CT	Surgery/histology
Curative resectability	8	6	10
Palliative resectability	13	7	16
Nonresectability	16	7	18

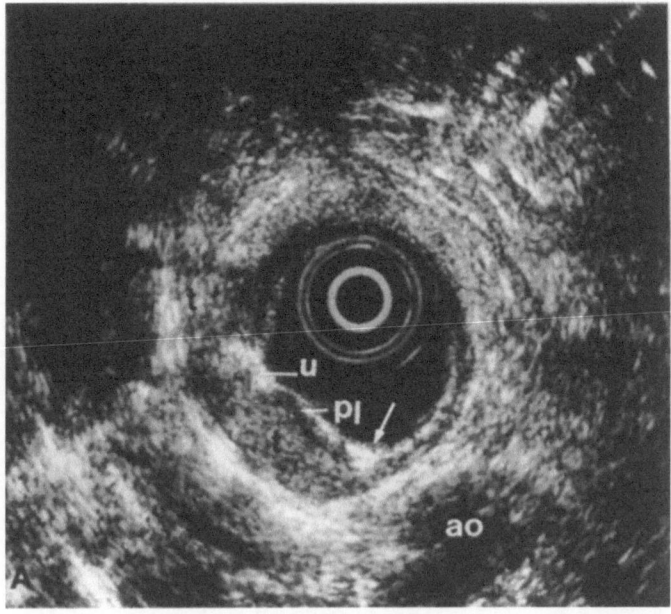

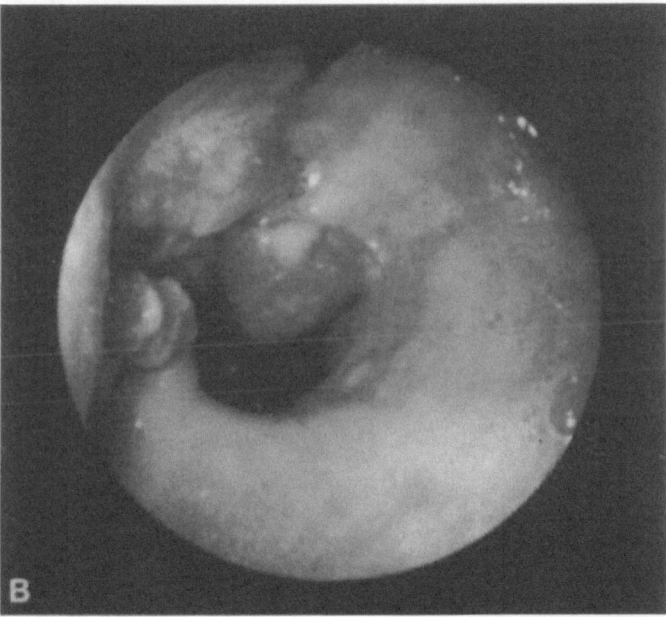

Fig. 1. A EUS image shows an ulcerative hypoechoic tumor mass *(t)* with polypoid margins *(pl)* penetrating into the adventitia and periesophageal fat tissue bordering the aorta *(ao)*. Note the clear transition between the normal and pathologic wall structure *(arrow)*. **B** Corresponding image of the polypoid esophageal carcinoma

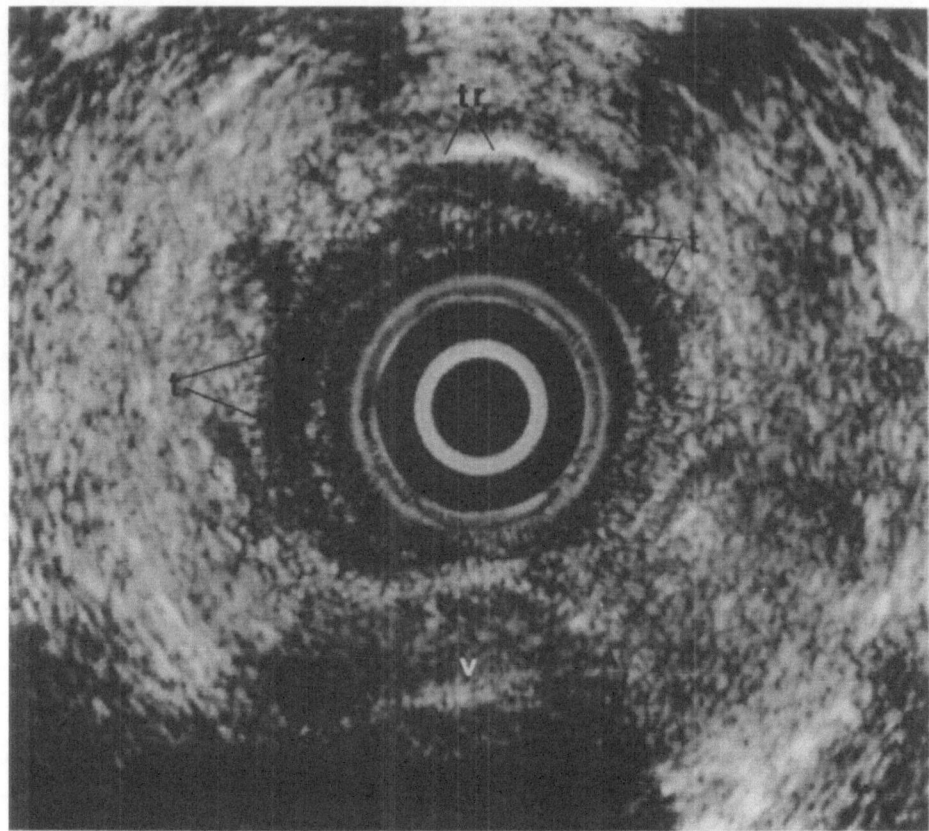

Fig. 2. EUS shows a circular hypoechoic transmural tumor mass *(t)* with deep penetration into the surrounding tissues. The trachea *(tr)* adjacent to the tumor mass is penetrated; *v*, vertebra

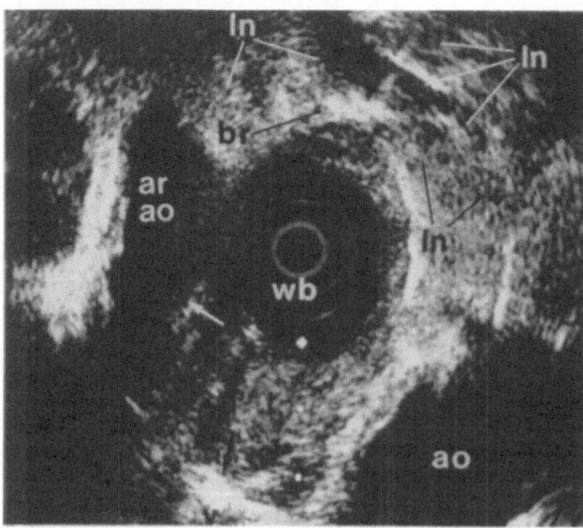

Fig. 4. EUS shows a hypoechoic tumor mass with deep penetration, particularly towards the vertebrae *(v) (black arrow)* and towards the aortic arch *(ar ao)*. *br,* Bronchus; *ln,* lymph nodes; *v,* vertebra

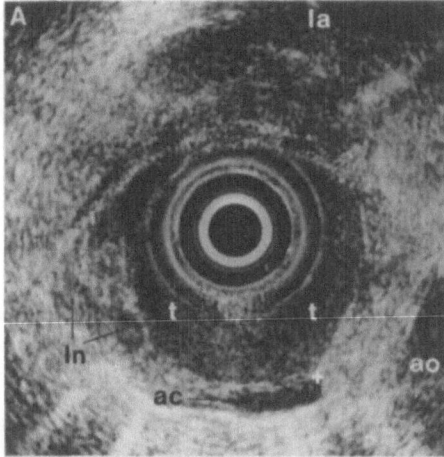

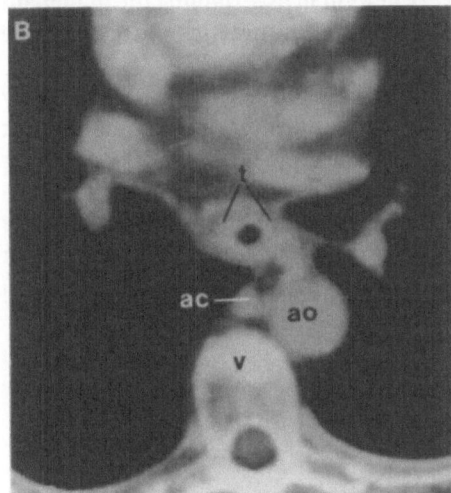

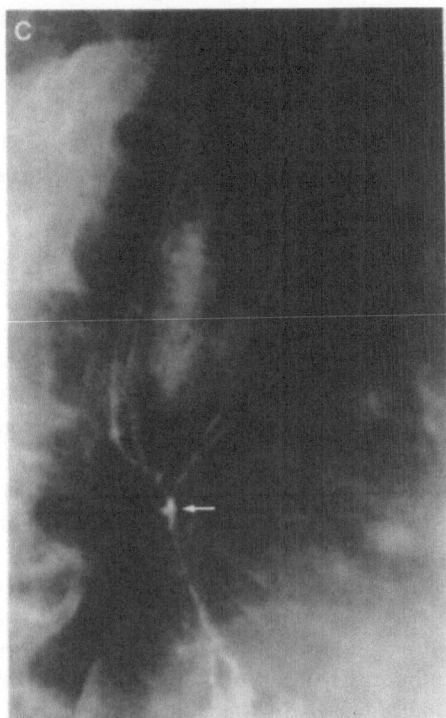

Fig. 3. A EUS image shows circular transmural hypoechoic structure with deep penetration into the surrounding periesophageal fat tissue bordering the azygos vein. *ao,* aorta; *la,* left atrium. **B** CT scan reveals thickening of the esophageal wall *(t)* bordering the azygos vein *(ac)* and aorta *(ao); v,* vertrebra. **C** Corresponding radiology image shows the stenosing esophageal carcinoma *(arrow)*

Gastric Tumor

EUS of the stomach is very valuable in the detection and staging of gastric neoplasm. When the lesion is found endoscopically, then the balloon and/or the lumen can be filled with water to visualize the longitudinal extent and the depth of infiltration together with adjacent lymph node abnormalities.

Benign Tumors

The most important benign lesion is a leiomyoma. Small leiomyomas have a homogeneous echopattern and sharply demarcated boundaries. Occasionally local thickening of the muscularis propria or even the muscularis mucosae can clearly be visualized, which is very helpful in making the diagnosis. Large leiomyomas may have an inhomogeneous echopattern because of the presence of blood vessels, ulcerative or necrotic lesions, or calcification within the tumor masses. The boundaries of lesions are sharply demarcated and compress but do not penetrate into the surrounding tissue. Extramural lesions compressing the gastric wall such as pancreatic pseudocyst, metastatic lymph nodes, fundic varices or aneurysm of the splenic artery, hepatomegaly or splenomegaly, ectopic pancreas, or Ménétrier's disease can easily be ruled out by EUS.

Malignant Tumors

The most common malignant submucosal lesions are leiomyosarcoma and leiomyoblastoma, which usually reveal an inhomogenous echopattern with the presence of a central ulcer or necrosis. Supplementary findings such as bizarre boundaries and the presence of suspicious lymph nodes may be very helpful in ascertaining the malignant character of the lesion. However, sharply demarcated boundaries do not exclude malignancy.

The most important and common gastric malignancy is a carcinoma. An early gastric carcinoma is visualized as a hypoechoic echopattern localized in the mucosa and/or submucosa with no penetration into the muscularis propria and with or without adjacent lymph node abnormalities. In contrast, an advanced gastric cancer is visualized as a hypoechoic intramural lesion with penetration into or through the muscularis propria and usually associated with lymph node abnormalities (Fig. 5). In

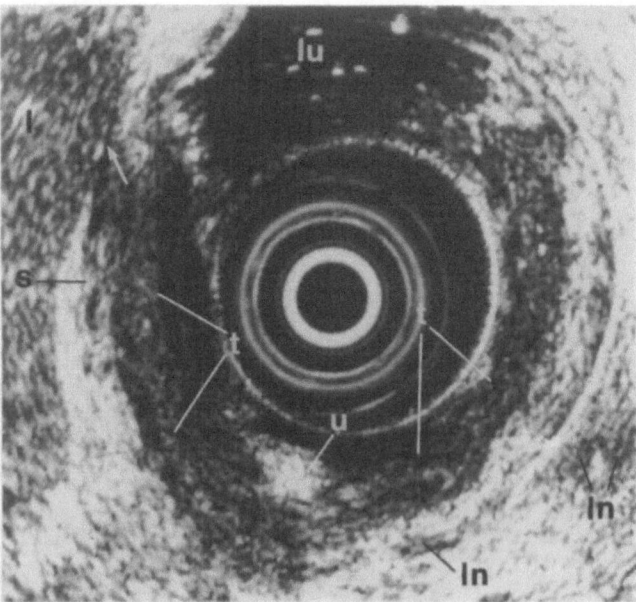

Fig. 5. EUS shows a hypoechoic echopattern with penetration into the serosal layer *(s)*, with some adjacent lymph nodes *(ln)* not suspicious of metastatic involvement. Note the unclear boundaries and more hyperechoic echopattern of the lymph nodes. *u*, ulcer; *lu*, lumen; *l*, liver

order to assess the accuracy and limitations of EUS in the preoperative assessment of resectability patients are divided into three groups:

- *Group 1* (Local curative resectability): EUS shows a clearly demarcated intramural hypoechoic lesion with no penetration through the organ boundaries (muscularis propria) and with or without adjacent lymph node abnormalities.

- *Group 2* (Palliative resectability): EUS shows a sharply demarcated hypoechoic tumor mass with no deep penetration into the surrounding tissue and usually with distant lymph node abnormalities.

- *Group 3* (Nonresectability): EUS shows deep penetration of a malignant lesion into the surrounding tissue, e. g., major blood vessels, hepatoduodenal ligament, and metastasis in the greater omentum or organs, e. g., pancreas, liver, and colon. In case of diffuse submucosal signet cell carcinoma of the stomach (linitis plastica) resection is usually not of benefit to the patient. Even though the malignancy is often locally resectable, the prognosis is still very poor (Fig. 6). Data collected in a

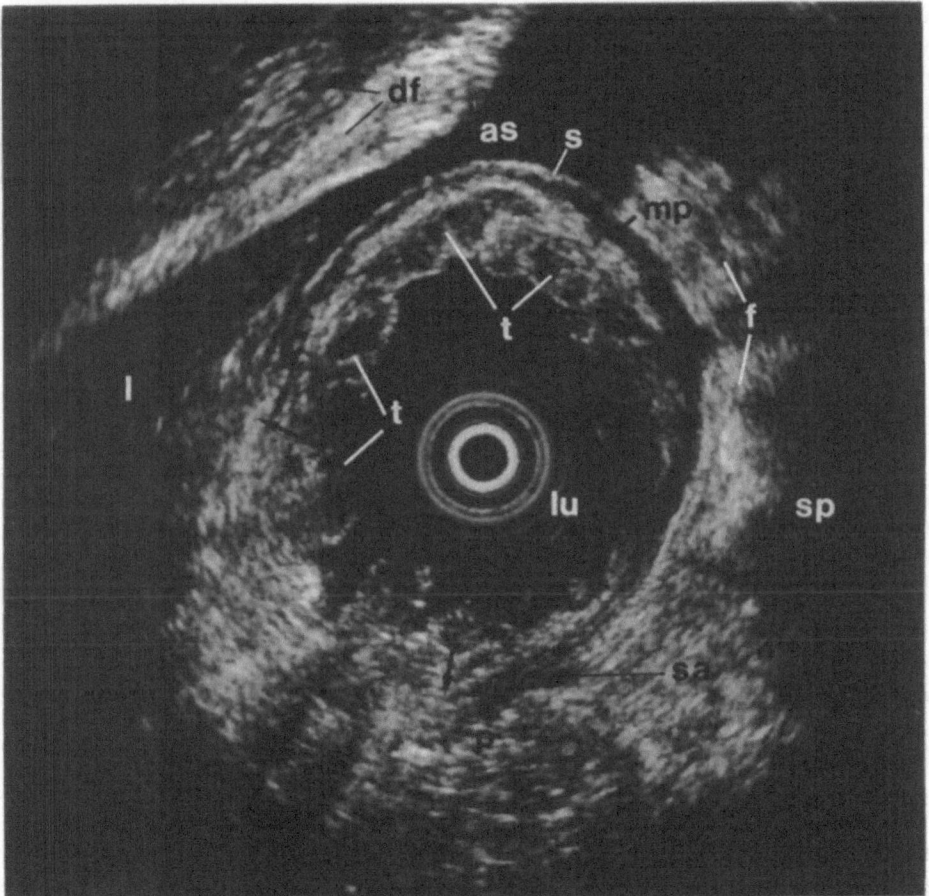

Fig. 6. EUS shows diffusely spreading hypoechoic tumor mass *(t)* localized in the submucosa with some penetration through the muscularis propria *(mp) (arrows)*. *as,* Ascites; *df,* diaphragm; *l,* liver; *p,* pancreas; *s,* serosa; *sp,* spleen, *sa,* splenic artery

Table 3. Summary of the results of EUS in assessing resectability of gastric carcinoma

	EUS correct diagnosis	Surgery/histology
Curative resectability	17	20
Palliative resectability	13	15
Nonresectability	14	17

prospective study and summarized in the Table 3 support these definitions of curative resectability, palliative resectability, and nonresectability.

Non-Hodgkin lymphoma of the stomach is recognized increasingly often. Major problems are often encountered in staging such lesions. EUS shows gastric non-Hodgkin lymphoma as a polypoid, ulcerative, or polypoid-ulcerative and/or diffuse transmural infiltration together with perigastric lymph node abnormalities [7]. Occasionally an extensive hypoechoic tumor mass immediately adjacent to the extensive ulcerative lesion can be identified. Difficulty may arise in case of giant folds associated with a gastric ulcer which may mimic a gastric non-Hodgkin lymphoma because of the similar transmural hypoechoic echopattern, especially when transmural infiltration together with an extensive ulcerative lesion is visualized. A difficulty with EUS is differentiating between inflammatory changes secondary to ulceration, either in the gastric wall or in lymph nodes. Therefore hypoechoic intramural changes and hypoechoic, sharply demarcated lymph nodes adjacent to an ulcerative lesion may be compatible with à benign lesion and do not automatically indicate malignancy. In the near future endosonographically guided biopsy or cytological puncture may solve such problems. When compared with CT, EUS appears superior in the assessment of resectability of gastric malignancy (Table 4).

Table 4. Summary of the results of EUS and CT scanning in assessing resectability of gastric carcinoma

	EUS	CT	Surgery/histology
Curative resectability	17	12	20
Palliative resectability	10	6	13
Nonresectability	13	7	15

Pancreatic Tumors

Benign Pancreatic Lesion Mimicking Pancreatic Malignancy

The most common benign pancreatic lesion mimicking pancreatic malignancy is a noncommunicating pancreatic pseudocyst obstructing the main pancreatic duct. By placing the echoprobe as close as possible to the obstructive ductular lesion, the distinction between a benign and malignant process can be made. Pancreatic pseudocysts are usually visualized as an anechoic structure with smooth contours, occasionally with some inhomogeneous echopattern. In contrast, pancreatic cancer is visualized as a hypoechoic inhomogeneous lesion with polycyclic or bizarre contours, usually associated with suspicious lymph nodes. Groove pancreatitis with irregular abnormalities of the common bile duct and/or of the pancreatic duct may strongly mimic pancreatic malignancy on ERCP. EUS allows visualization of the ductular abnormality and the presence of a hypoechoic echopattern between the duodenal wall and the pancreas, whereas the pancreatic parenchyma does not suggest malignant transformation.

Pancreatic Cancer

The transduodenal and transgastric approach allows clear visualization of the pancreas and the distal part of the biliary tract. A pancreatic carcinoma is visualized as a hypoechoic, sharply or bizarrely demarcated parenchymal echopattern which often appears more hypoechoic than the surrounding tissues. The parenchymal and ductular abnormalities together with the peripancreatic lymph nodes can readily be seen. Supplementary findings such as compression of the pancreatic duct, bile duct, or both, and prestenotic dilatation corresponding to the ERCP findings of a double duct are also very helpful in detecting the malignant nature of the lesion.

Resectability for cure is determined by the presence of a hypoechoic pancreatic lesion with a more hypoechoic echopattern than the surrounding tissue together with the absence of penetration into the surrounding blood vessels or adjacent lymph nodes (Fig. 7). Intraductular carcinoma, usually multilocated, is visualized as a hypoechoic intraductular lesion originating from the ductural wall. Although the tumors are locally resectable the prognosis of such a lesion is dubious. A clearly demarcated hypoechoic tumor mass without penetration into the adjacent major blood vessels but with evidence of lymph node involvement indicates the palliative character of the surgical resection. Pancreatic cancer is considered nonresectable when there is deep penetration into the surrounding tissues and/or the major blood vessels such as the mesenteric artery, celiac trunk, aorta, vena cava, or splenoportal confluence (Fig. 8). Visualization of the retroperitoneal area is essential for the determination of nonresectability. Occasionally an extensive anechoic cavity compatible with a necrotic mass can be visualized immediately adjacent to the main lesion. This also indicates nonresectability (Fig. 9). Liver metastasis prohibits curative resection [9, 12]. Data collected in the Table 5 support the value of EUS in defining the curative resectability, palliative resectability, or nonresectability of a pancreatic carcinoma.

Table 5. Summary of the results of EUS in assessing resectability of pancreatic carcinoma

	EUS	Surgery/histology
Curative	2	3
Palliative	10	11
Nonresectability	5	7

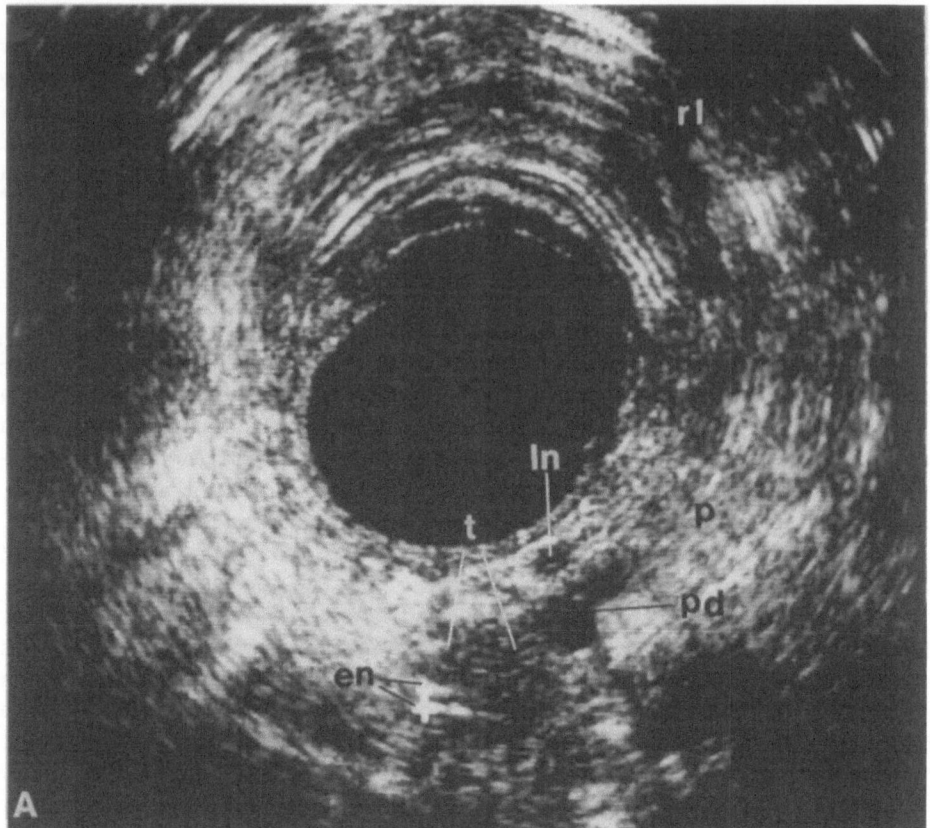

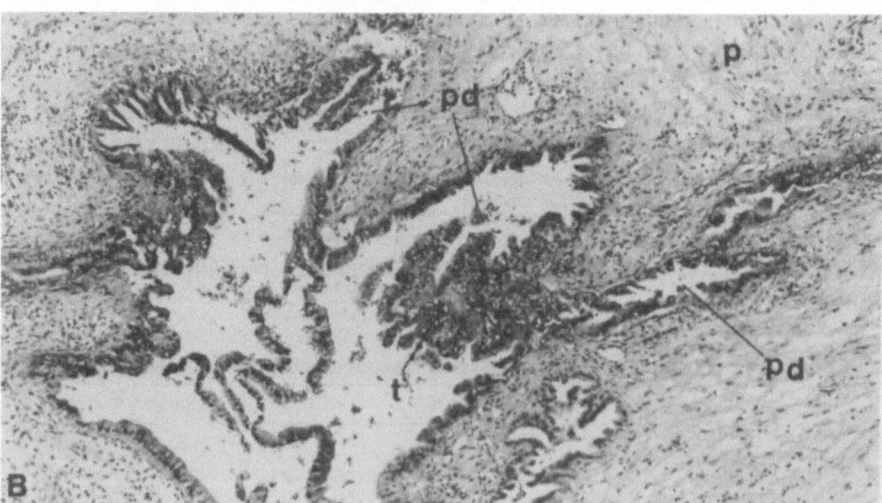

Fig. 7. A EUS shows a circumscribed hypoechoic tumor *(t)* containing the endoprosthesis *(en)* bordering the pancreatic duct *(pd)* with a small lymph node *(ln)* proven to be negative for metastasis by histology. **B** Corresponding histology of the resection specimen revealing an intraductular carcinoma *(t)* of the pancreas *(p); pd,* pancreatic duct

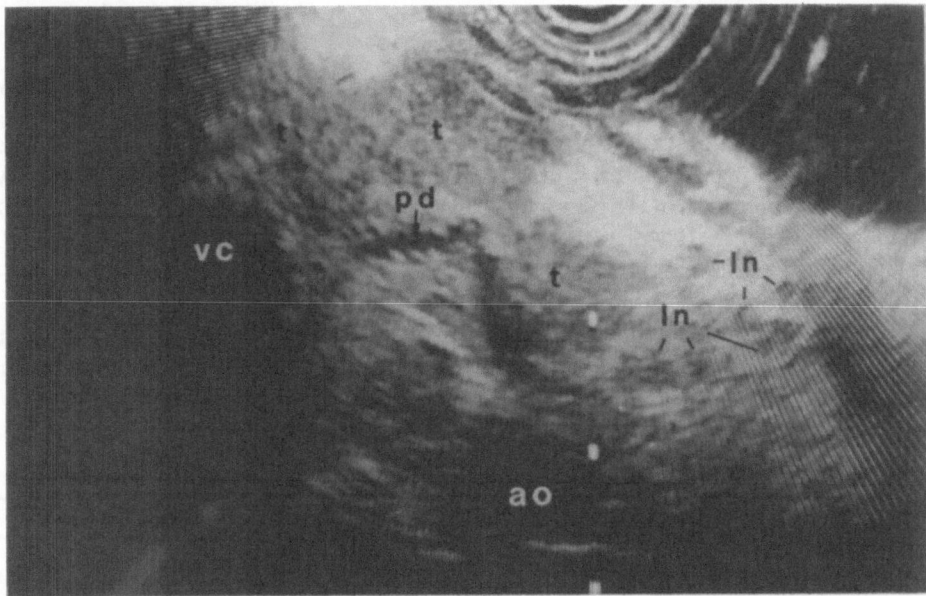

Fig. 8. EUS shows a hypoechoic pancreatic tumor mass *(t)* with clearly demarcated boundaries with compression of the pancreatic duct *(pd)*. Note the retroperitoneal spread of the tumor mass near the aorta *(ao)* and vena cava *(vc); ln,* lymph nodes

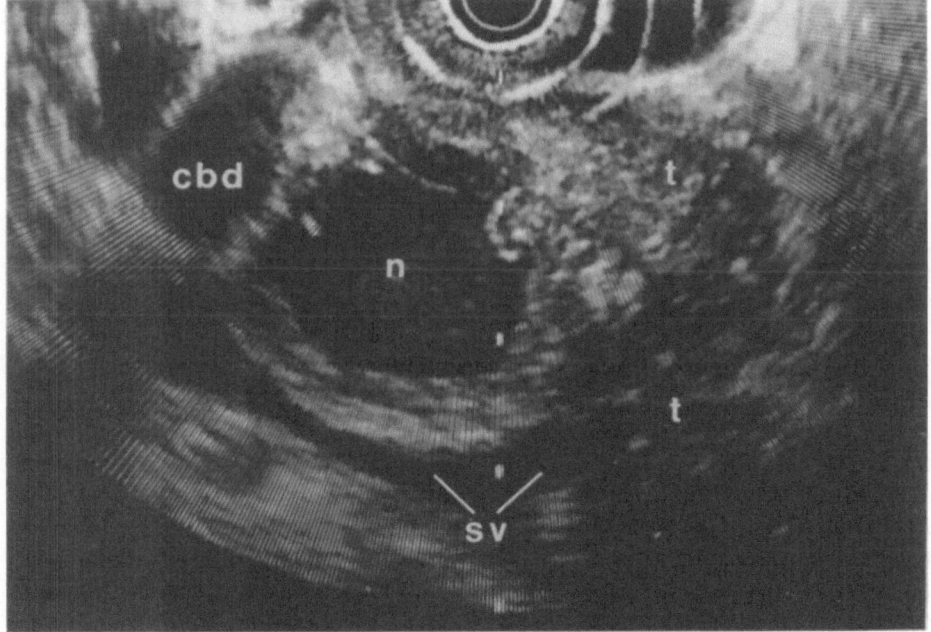

Fig. 9. EUS picture shows an inhomogeneous tumor mass *(t)* with an adjacent necrotic cavity *(n)* compressing the common bile duct *(cbd)*. Note the penetration to the splenic vein *(sv)*

Peripapillary Tumor

A peripapillary tumor is visualized as a hypoechoic intramural lesion immediately adjacent to the peripapillary common bile duct and/or the pancreatic duct. Differentiation between adenomamyomatosis and carcinoma is difficult or impossible, except when evidence of penetration into or through the muscularis propria is lacking. A polypoid configuration of the tumor can clearly be seen by rapidly filling the duodenal lumen with water and by directly approaching the lesion with ultrasonic beam [5, 9, 12]. In advanced peripapillary cancer, invasion into the adjacent pancreatic parenchyma can clearly be visualized, which may make the differentiation between pancreatic cancer and peripapillary carcinoma difficult. Data collected in Table 6 support the value of EUS in assessing the curative resectability, palliative resectability, or nonresectability of pancreatic cancer.

Table 6. Summary of the results of EUS in assessing resectability of peripapillary carcinoma

	EUS correct diagnosis	Surgery/histology
Curative resectability	7	9
Palliative resectability	2	3
Nonresectability	2	2

Distal Common Bile Duct Lesion

Malignancy in the distal common bile duct is visualized as a polypoid hypoechoic structure originating from the bile duct wall and protruding into the dilated lumen. After insertion of a biliary endoprosthesis, a hypoechoic tumor structure containing a hyperechoic line is characteristic of bile duct malignancy. An endoprosthesis is sometimes a useful guide for localizing the main lesion and does not prohibit accurate visualization of the lesion (Fig. 10).

Local curative resectability can be confidently diagnosed when the tumor is sharply demarcated without or with regional lymph node involvement. A locally resectable tumor with multiple regional and distant suspicious lymph nodes is highly suggestive of the palliative character of the resection. Bile duct malignancy with deep penetration into the adjacent pancreas can often cause difficulties with respect to differentiation from a pancreatic carcinoma. The presence of pancreatic duct abnormality is more characteristic of pancreatic carcinoma than of bile duct malignancy. Evidence of nonresectability can be obtained on the basis of penetration of the tumor into the adjacent major blood vessels, e. g., the hepatic artery, the portal vein, the celiac trunc, the aorta, or the vena cave, and/or metastasis to the liver [9, 12]. The topographic anatomical relationship between the papilla of Vater, the distal common bile duct, and the pancreatic duct may at times make exact identification of the origin of the tumor difficult. Endosonographically guided puncture will further enhance the value of EUS. Data collected in Table 7 support the value of EUS in defining the curative resectability, palliative resectability, or nonresectability of a common bile duct carcinoma.

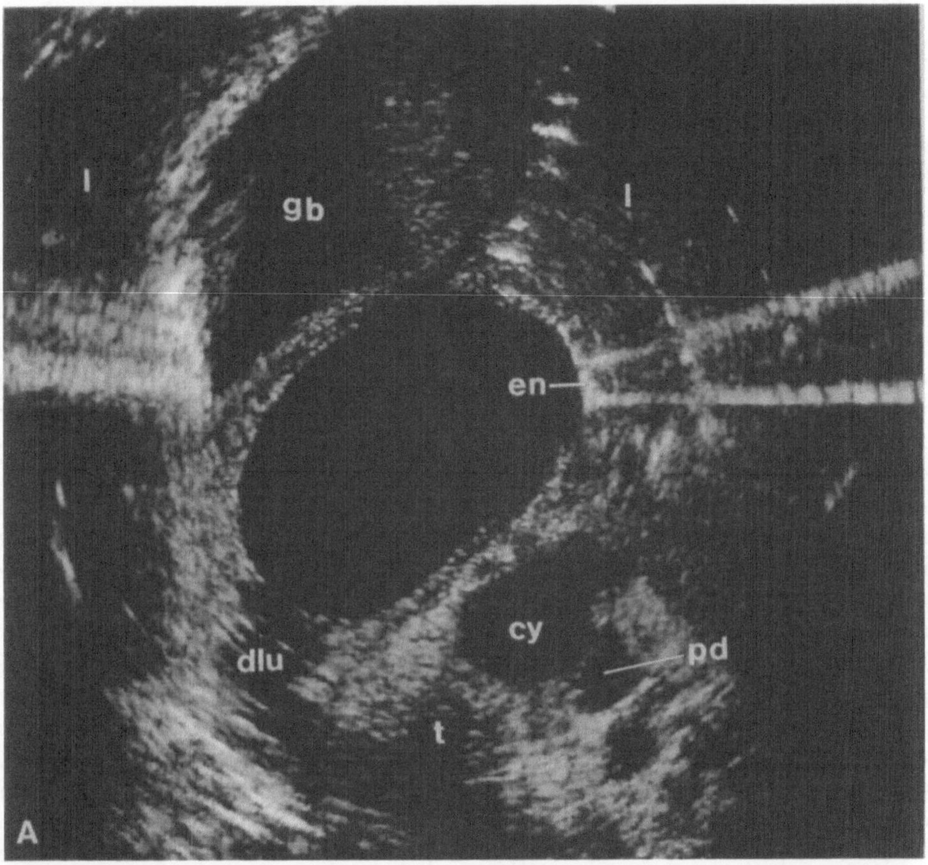

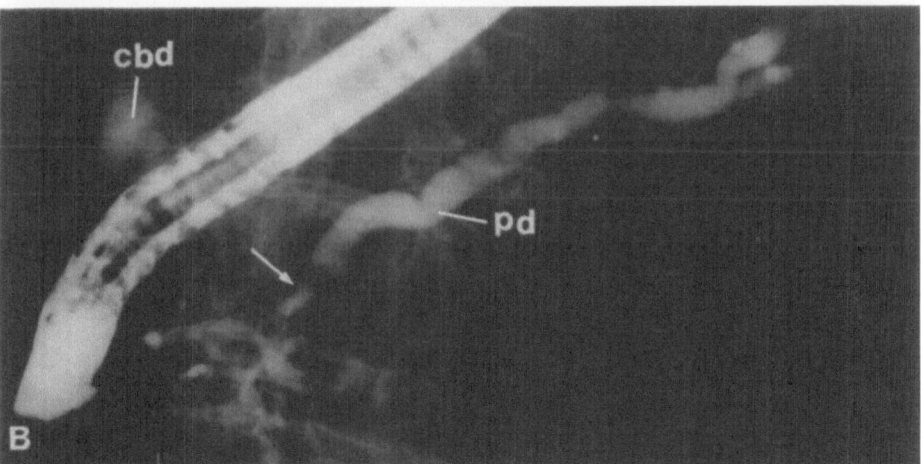

Fig. 10. A EUS shows a circumscribed hypoechoic tumor *(t)* with an adjacent cystic lesion *(cy)* compressing the pancreatic duct *(pd)*. *dlu*, Duodenal lumen; *l*, liver; *en*, biliary endoprosthesis; *gb*, gallbladder. **B** Corresponding ERCP image shows the dilated common bile duct *(cbd)* and some irregularity of the adjacent pancreatic duct *(arrow)*; *pd*, pancreatic duct

Table 7. Summary of the results of EUS in assessing resectability of distal common bile duct carcinoma

	EUS correct diagnosis	Surgery/histology
Curative resection	4	6
Palliative resection	8	11
Nonresectability	2	2

Tumor of the Hepatobiliary Bifurcation (Klatskin Tumor)

The biliary tree can be recognized by slowly withdrawing the instrument from the area of the papilla of Vater and using the typical localization of the common bile duct immediately adjacent to the duodenal wall as a landmark. From the apical bulbar scanning position the liver hilum and the gallbladder can be visualized. The confluence of the hepatic duct in the porta hepatis is usually readily recognizable. A malignancy is usually visualized as a hypoechoic intraductular structure localized immediately adjacent to the bifurcation of the bile duct together with dilatation of the intrahepatic ducts and a normal-caliber distal common bile duct. A clearly demarcated intraductal lesion localized only in one liver lobe without penetration into the adjacent liver and the portal vein is indicative of local curative resectability. A hypoechoic tumor mass extending into both the adjacent liver lobes with local penetration into the portal vein, and multiple suspicious lymph nodes is strongly suggestive of thè palliative nature of the procedure. Deep penetration of a hypoechoic tumor mass into the adjacent major blood vessels, e. g., portal vein or hepatic artery, or multiple liver metastasis are considered to indicate nonresectability [9, 12]. Data collected in Table 8 support the value of EUS in defining the curative and palliative resectability of a Klatskin tumor. Follow-up investigation after liver resection is accurate and essential because both lymph node abnormality and/or intraductal tumor recurrence can readily be visualized. This is of utmost importance since ERCP is usually technically impossible after hepaticojejunostomy. Conventional ultrasonography and CT are considerably less accurate in the detection of such recurrent malignancies.

Table 8. Summary of the results of EUS in assessing resectability of a Klatskin tumor

	EUS correct diagnosis	Surgery/histology
Curative resection	2	3
Palliative resection	12	12

Gallbladder Malignancy

Carcinoma of the gallbladder is visualized as a hypoechoic polypoid tumor structure originating from the wall or protruding into the cavity of the gallbladder (Fig. 11). In advanced stages tumor extension along the hepatic duct into the hepatobiliary bifurcation can be recognized. In such cases differentiation between a Klatskin tumor and a

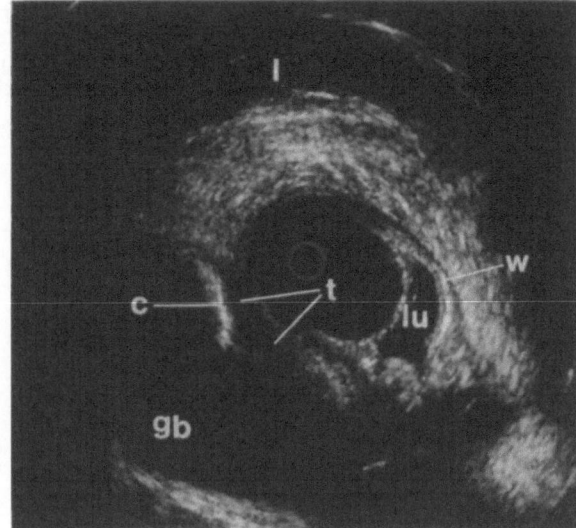

Fig. 11. EUS shows a hypoechoic tumor mass *(t)* in the wall of the gallbladder *(gb)* with some penetration near the adjacent duodenal lumen *(lu)*. *w,* Normal duodenal wall on the contralateral side; *c,* concrement in the gallbladder; *l,* right lobe of the liver

gallbladder carcinoma is often very difficult or even impossible. Hydrops of the gallbladder due to primary cholangiocarcinoma can readily be differentiated from concrements in the cystic duct such as are seen in the Mirrizzi syndrome. Evidence of nonresectability is based on deep penetration of the malignancy into the surrounding tissues or the adjacent liver parenchyma. An extensive hypoechoic tumor mass of the gallbladder with penetration into the adjacent gastroduodenal wall with or without lymph node metastasis in the pancreatic head may mimic pancreatic cancer or groove pancreatitis. However, supplementary findings such as compression of the pancreatic duct with prestenotic dilatation or compression of both the pancreatic duct and the common bile duct, compatible with a double duct lesion as found by ERCP, may be very helpful in distinguishing malignancy in the gallbladder from cancer of the pancreas. An endosonographically guided cytological puncture or biopsy may help in ascertaining the malignant nature of such lesions.

References

1. Di Magno EP, Regan PT, Clain JE, James EM, Buxton JL (1982) Human endoscopic ultrasonography. Gastroenterology 83: 824–829
2. Lux G, Heyder N, Demling L (1982) Endoscopic ultrasonography – technique, orientation and diagnostic possibilities. Endoscopy 4: 220–225
3. Heyder N, Luth H, Lux G (1983) Ultraschalldiagnostik via Gastroskop. Ultraschall Med 4: 84–93
4. Strohm WD, Classen M (1984) Endosonographie mit einem Gastrofiberskop. Ultraschall Med 5: 84–93
5. Tio TL, Tytgat GNJ (1984) Endoscopic ultrasonography in the assessment of intra- and transmural infiltration of tumours in the oesophagus, stomach and papilla of Vater and in the detection of extraoesophageal lesions. Endoscopy 4: 220–225
6. Caletti G, Bolondi L, Brocchi P et al. (1983) Staging of gastric cancer by means of endoscopic ultrasonography (abstract). Gastroenterology 84: 13 866

7. Tio TL, den Hartog Jager FCA, Tytgat GNJ (1986) Endoscopic ultrasonography of Non-Hodgkin lymphoma of the stomach. Gastroenterology 91: 401–408
8. Tio TL, den Hartog Jager FCA, Tytgat GNJ (1986) The role of endoscopic ultrasonography in assessing local resectability of oesophagogastric malignancies. Scand J Gastroenterol (suppl 123) 21: 78–86
9. Tio TL, Tytgat GNJ (1986) Atlas of transintestinal ultrasonography. Mur Kostverloren BV, Aalsmeer, The Netherlands
10. Scand J Gastroenterol (1984) (suppl 102) 19: 5–37
11. Scand J Gastroenterol (1984) (suppl 94) 19: 1–106
12. Scand J Gastroenterol (1986) (suppl 123) 21: 1–169

XI Non-Hodgkin Lymphoma of the Stomach

Endosonography versus Computed Tomography, Endoscopy, and Histology

Introduction

The stomach is the predominant site of gastrointestinal (GI) non-Hodgkin lymphoma (NHL) [1–5]. Endoscopy allows three distinct patterns to be distinguished: diffuse infiltration, irregular ulceration, and a predominantly polypoid pattern [5]. The preliminary diagnosis cannot always be confirmed by endoscopic biopsies because the lesion arises from the lymphatic tissue, which may not be reached with a biopsy forceps [6, 7]. Computed tomography (CT) is frequently disappointing because of failure to characterize the GI wall involvement and lymph node abnormality [8–10]. Endoscopic ultrasonography (EUS) – a combination of two high technologies – is considered accurate in analyzing the GI wall and periintestinal lymph node abnormalities by directly approaching the target lesion with a high-frequency real-time echoprobe head via the intestinal lumen [11–18]. The aim of this study was to assess the accuracy and limitations of EUS

a) in diagnosing and staging according to the modified Ann-Arbor staging system (Table 1) [19], and

b) in follow-up of gastric NHL after treatment.

Table 1. Staging system in non-Hodgkin lymphoma of the stomach: modification of the Ann-Arbor staging

Stage	
I	Process limited to the stomach wall
II_1	The same as I with adjacent lymph node involvement
II_2	The same as II_1 with regional abdominal lymph node involvement
IIE	Local extension into surrounding (extralymphatic) organ
III	Involvement of lymph nodes above the diaphragm and/or of the spleen
IV	Involvement of various organs, such as lung parenchyma, liver, bone marrow, kidney, and skin

Materials and Methods

Between April 1984 and December 1987 EUS was performed in 31 patients with suspected or proven NHL of the stomach. The patients were divided into two groups. The first group consisted of nine patients in whom the diagnosis was confirmed at surgery ($n = 7$) or autopsy ($n = 2$). The indications for surgery were bleeding or

Table 2. The results of EUS, CT, and histology of the resection or autopsy specimens in the staging according to the modified Ann-Arbor system (group 1)

No. of Patients	Stage	EUS	CT	Histology	EUS follow-up
1	I	+	−	surgery	no
2	I	+	−	surgery	no
3	II	+	−	surgery	early gastric cancer
4	II	+	−	surgery	complete remission
5	II	+	no	surgery	no
6	III	+	+	autopsy	−
7	IV	−	+	surgery	no
8	IV	+	+	autopsy	−
9	IV	−	−	surgery	no

+, Correct interpretation by the imaging technique, as indicated by the histopathology
−, Incorrect interpretation by the imaging technique, as indicated by the histopathology

obstruction. In two patients follow-up EUS was performed (Table 2). There were four men and five women with ages ranging from 46 to 76 years. The second group consisted of 22 patients who did not undergo surgery. They were evaluated only with endoscopy and multiple biopsies. EUS was performed before and after radiotherapy or chemotherapy. There were 12 men and 10 women with ages ranging from 15 to 72 years. The diagnosis of NHL was considered using EUS if there was destruction of the normal gastric wall structure and submucosal or transmural infiltration with or without penetration into surrounding tissues, with or without perigastric lymph node abnormalities. Assessment of EUS accuracy was by comparison with the histology of multiple endoscopic biopsies or of the resected specimen when available.

The method of examination has been described elsewhere [11, 18]. Filling the gastric lumen with water facilitated clear visualization of the wall of the body and antrum of the stomach. The region of the cardia and pylorus was examined using a water-filled balloon attached to the transducer to optimize contact with the mucosa, while air accumulation between the transducer und mucosa was avoided. All studies were performed with a prototype or a commercially available Olympus echoendoscope (EU-M1 or EU-M2). The frequency of the transducer was 7.5 MHz and it had a penetration depth of approximately 10 cm and an optimal (theoretical) axial resolution of 0.2 mm. In later patients EUS was performed with a prototype Olympus echoendoscope with a frequency of 10 MHz. The penetration depth of this instrument is approximately 5 cm with an axial resolution of 0.1 mm. Complications were not encountered in this study.

Results

Table 2 summarizes the results of EUS, CT, histology of the resection specimens, and follow-up (group 1). Stage I disease was diagnosed when a limited hypoechoic intramural echopattern without evidence of lymph node involvement was found ($n = 2$) (Fig. 1). Stage II disease was diagnosed when a transmural hypoechoic lesion

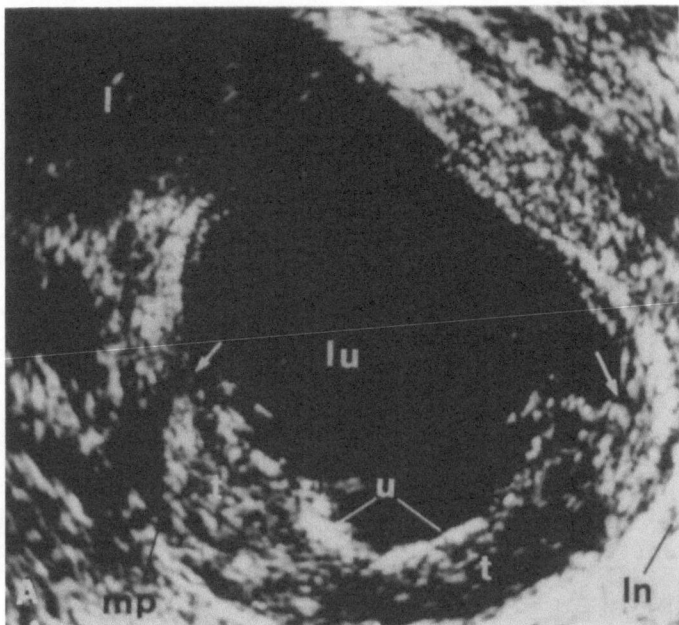

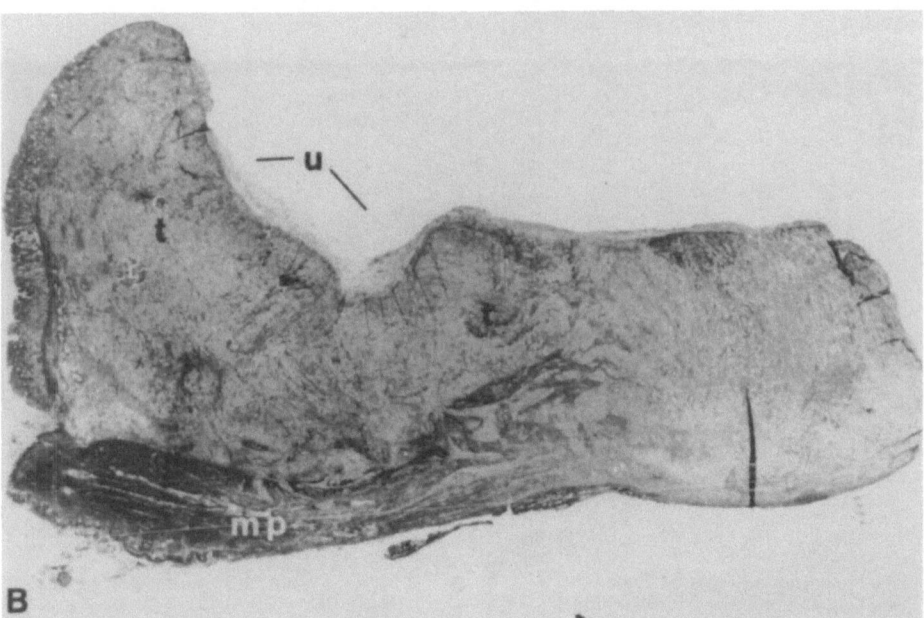

Fig. 1. A EUS shows a clearly demarcated hypoechoic lesion *(t)* directly adjacent to an ulcerative lesion *(u)* with penetration into the muscularis propria *(mp)* and a hypoechoic, unclearly delineated lymph node not suspicious of malignancy. Note the clear transition between the normal and pathologic wall structure *(arrows); l, liver.* **B** Corresponding histology of the resected specimen shows a NHL infiltration adjacent to an ulcer with penetration into the muscularis propria. The resemblance between the EUS picture and the corresponding histology is obvious

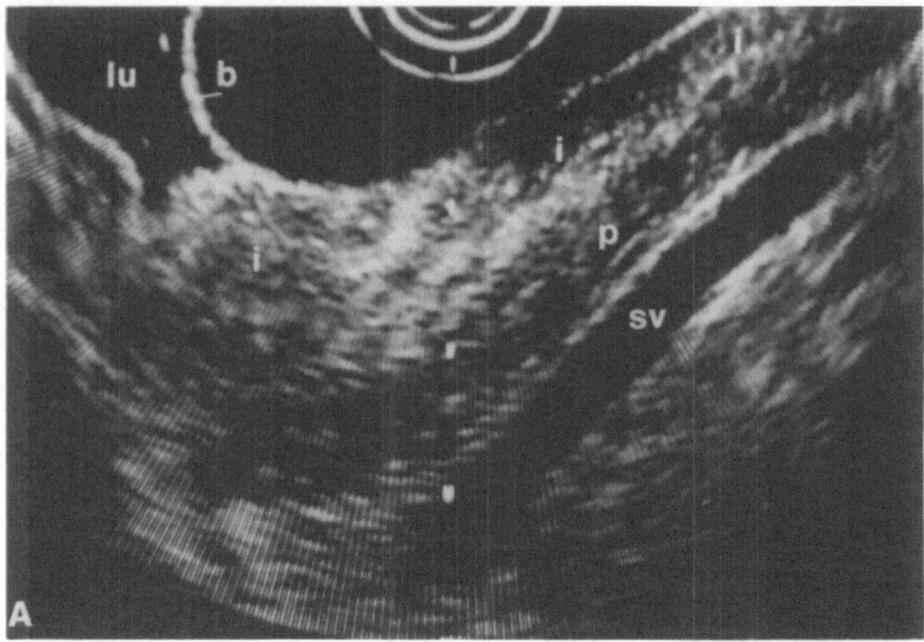

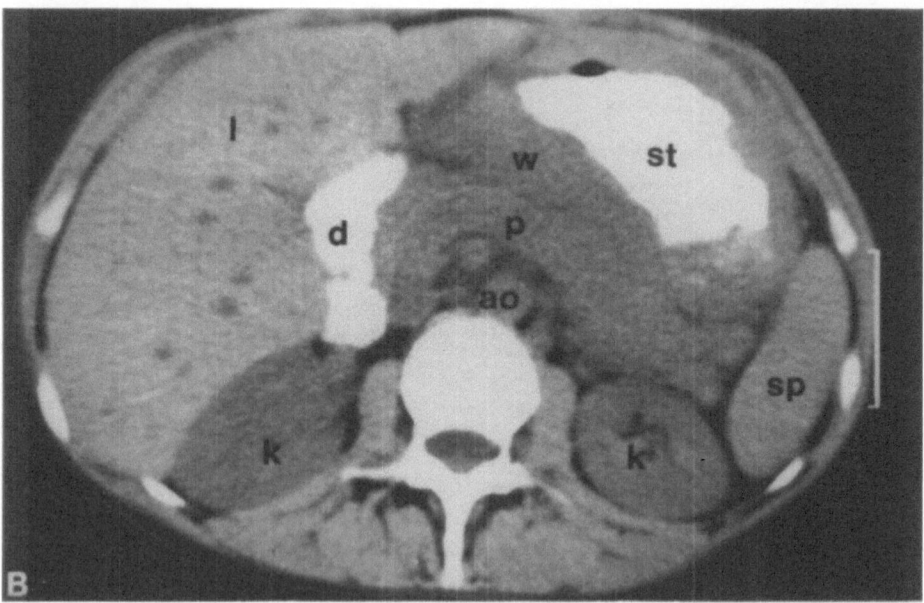

Fig. 2. A EUS shows a clearly demarcated hypoechoic tumor *(t)* adjacent to an ulcerative lesion *(u)*. Note the clear transition between the normal and pathologic wall structure *(arrow)*. *m*, Mucosa; *sm*, submucosa; *m*, muscularis propria; *s*, subserosa-serosa. **B** Corresponding CT image shows a thickening of the gastric wall *(w)* adjacent to the pancreas *(p)*. *st*, stomach lumen; *d*, duodenal lumen; *k*, kidney; *sp*, spleen; *l*, liver

without ($n = 1$) or with local penetration in continuity with the pancreas ($n = 1$) or the left liver lobe ($n = 1$) together with involved adjacent lymph nodes was visualized. The EUS findings were confirmed by histology of the resection specimen or at surgery (Fig. 2). CT did not show the mural and nodal abnormalities. Stage III disease was correctly diagnosed by EUS and CT based upon infiltration into the spleen ($n = 1$), which was confirmed by autopsy. In contrast, stage IV disease was misdiagnosed using EUS in two out of three patients because the retroperitoneal lymph node abnormalities and the infiltration into the right lobe ($n = 2$) of the liver could not visualized, either because the pylorus could not be passed by the endoscope or because the duodenum could not be reached due to Billroth II stomach resection. Moreover, the gastric wall structure was not clearly visualized because the lumen was not adequately filled with water. Diagnoses using CT were correct in two of three patients. Complete remission was diagnosed using EUS during follow-up after chemo- or radiotherapy. EUS showed when mural and nodal abnormalities disappeared, as occurred in two patients with stage II disease, in both of whom lesions had previously proven to be nonresectable at surgery. However, during further evaluation, approximately 18 months later, EUS showed in one of these patients, a limited hypoechoic submucosal lesion underneath a superficial ulcer in the more distal part of the stomach. Endoscopic biopsies resulted in the diagnosis of adenocarcinoma. Histology of the gastrectomy specimen showed early gastric carcinoma and no evidence of remaining lymphoma.

Table 3 summarizes the results of endoscopy and EUS before and after treatment (group 2). Three endoscopic patterns reported in a previous study [5] were also visualized with EUS as well. At endoscopy the diffusely infiltrating malignancy was considered to be an extensive ($n = 1$) or a limited ($n = 2$) infiltration. In these patients EUS showed a hypoechoic diffuse transmural infiltration penetrating deeply into the pancreas with adjacent lymph node involvement and associated with ascites ($n = 1$), or a limited hypoechoic submucosal infiltration beyond the nodular mucosal deformity without evidence of deep penetration or lymph node involvement ($n = 2$)

Table 3. A comparison of endoscopy and EUS before and after chemo- and/or radiotherapy (group 2)

No. of patients	Endoscopy			EUS		
	Initial	Follow-up		Initial	Follow-up	
		PR	CR		PR	CR
3	Diffuse infiltration	Reduction of gross pathology	Disappearance	Diffuse transmural infiltration, LN. abn.	Reduction mural + LN. abn.	Reappearance of 5 layers + LN. abn.
15	Ulcers	Reduction, partial healing	Healing	Intramural hypoechoic lesions	Reduction	Reappearance of mural + LN. abn.
4	Polypoid lesions	Reduction	Disappearance	Intramural hypoechoic lesions + LN. abn.	Reduction of depth of infiltration + LN. abn.	Disappearance of mural + LN. abn.

PR, Partial remission; CR, complete remission; LN. abn., lymph node abnormalities

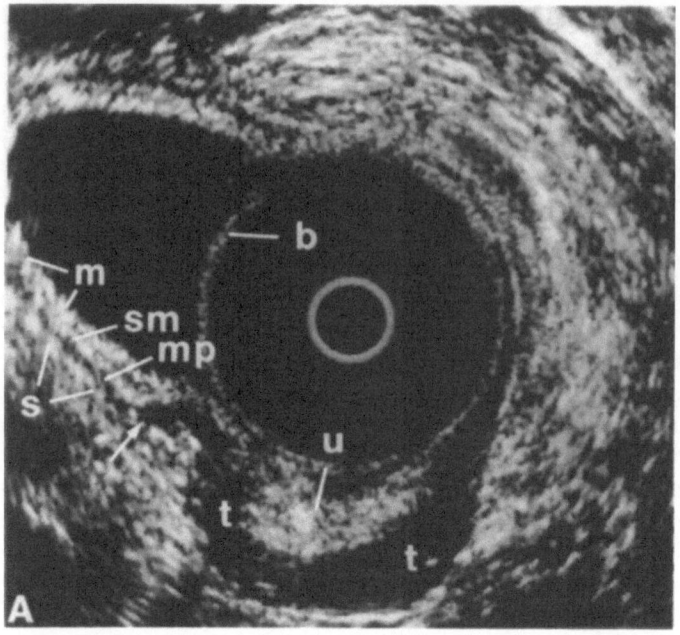

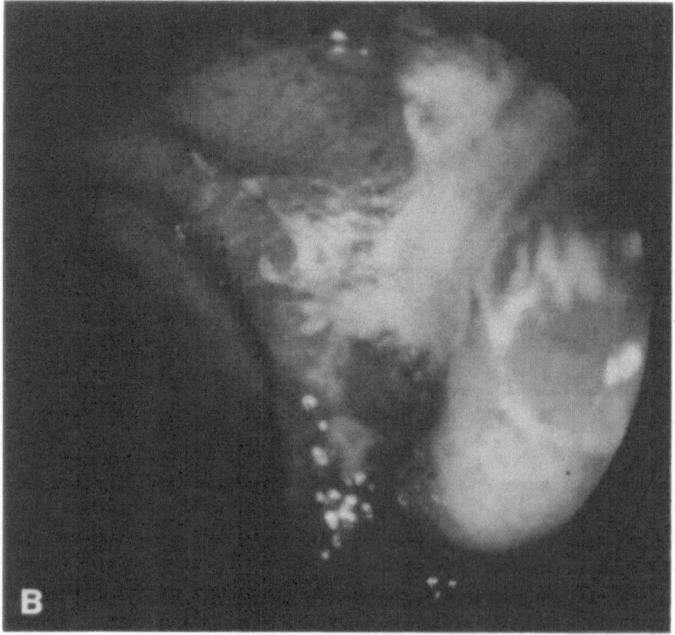

Fig. 3. A EUS shows a hypoechoic transmural infiltration *(i)* adjacent to the pancreas *(p)*. *sv,* Splenic vein; *lu,* gastric lumen. **B** Endoscopy shows an ulcerative lesion with some nodular margins

(Fig. 3). With respect to the ulcerative type, endoscopy showed either small flat ulcers ($n = 4$) or extensive ulcerative lesions ($n = 11$). Either transmurally deeply infiltrating abnormalities with somewhat polypoid margins ($n = 11$) or limited hypoechoic echopatterns ($n = 4$) immediately adjacent to an ulcerous defect (Fig. 4) were visualized with EUS. At endoscopy small ($n = 2$) or extensive bulging lesions were found ($n = 2$). EUS showed a limited intramural hypoechoic echopattern adjacent to a small polypoid bulge ($n = 2$) or a transmural hypoechoic abnormality beyond an extensive bulge ($n = 2$) (Fig. 5).

At endoscopy partial remission was defined as a reduction of the extent of mucosal abnormalities or of the depth of ulcerative lesions. EUS showed partial remission as a reduction of the intramural hypoechoic abnormality and a decrease in size and number of lymph nodes. Complete remission was documented at endoscopy when the mucosal abnormalities disappeared and multiple biopsies were negative for NHL infiltration. Complete remission was documented with EUS when mural lymph abnormalities and abnormal lymph nodes disappeared completely.

Discussion

As illustrated in the figures and Table 2, staging of gastric NHL according to the modified Ann-Arbor classification can be carried out quite accurately with EUS. This is based upon the ability to visualize the intramural extent and depth of infiltration together with the detection of perigastrointestinal lymph node involvement. EUS appears to be superior to CT because of more clear visualization of the local malignant penetration into the surrounding tissues or organs such as the pancreas, spleen, and adjacent liver lobes. A distinction between lymph nodes and blood vessels can readily be made with EUS because of its real-time properties. As a rule, malignant lymph nodes in continuity with a mural abnormality exhibit a similar echopattern to the mural malignancy and nearly always have clearly demarcated boundaries [14–16]. In contrast, CT scanning does not always allow clear differentiation between blood vessels and lymph nodes because of its static nature. The primary lesion can be distinguished from the surrounding tissue because of the more hypoechoic appearance and the disruption of the normal layering pattern of the stomach wall [15, 16]. The transition between normal and pathologic wall structure in both cross and longitudinal sections can be distinguished with EUS because of the ability to image the gastrointestinal wall in detail and to maneuver the transducer endoscopically. CT scanning may show gastric wall abnormalities only as thickening of the wall. Moreover, only cross sections can be obtained. Therefore, stages I and II can only be distinguished accurately with EUS. In contrast, CT scanning is more accurate in the assessment of stage IV because involvement of distant lymph nodes and infiltration into various organs such as the right lobe of the liver can usually be recognized. EUS has limitations in ascertaining stage IV because of the limited penetration depth of ultrasound and because of the difficulty in reaching the target lesion both endoscopically and sonographically. EUS appears superior when compared to endoscopy alone, as endoscopy only enables the intraluminal, or in fact the intramural, extent of the malignancy to be visualized but not the depth of infiltration or the adjacent lymph node involvement. Infiltration beneath normal overlying mucosa can only be recog-

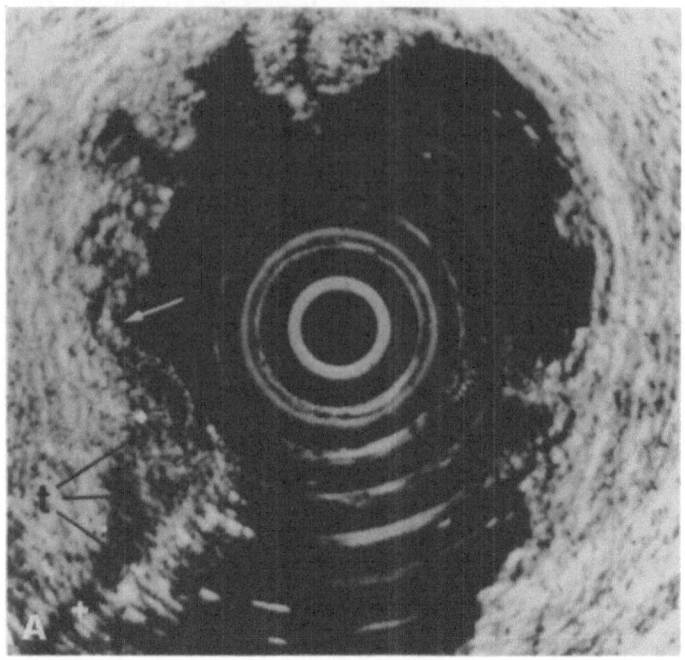

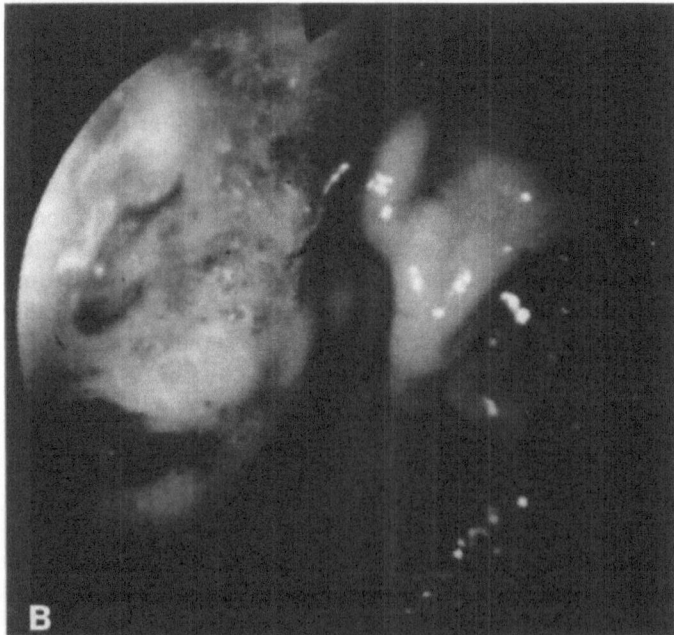

Fig. 4. A EUS shows a clearly demarcated hypoechoic lesion immediately adjacent to a small polypoid lesion *(arrow)*. **B** Endoscopy shows a small polypoid lesion *(arrow)*

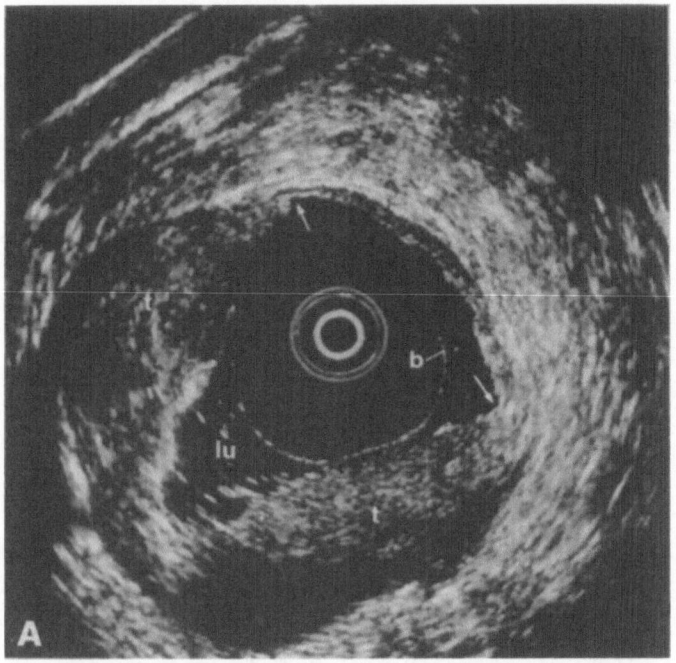

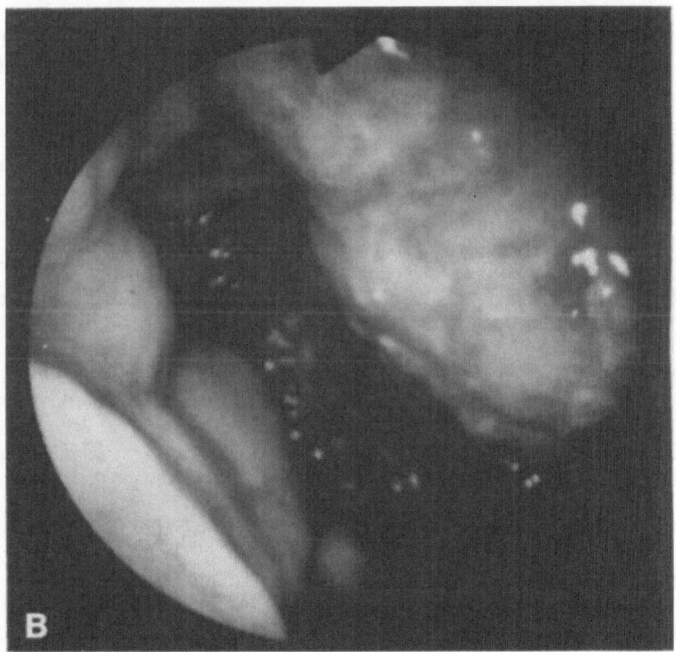

Fig. 5. A EUS shows clearly demarcated hypoechoic tumors *(t)* causing extensive polypoid lesions. Note the clear transition between the normal and pathologic wall structure *(arrows); lu,* gastric lumen. **B** Corresponding macroscopy shows extensive polypoid lesions in the proximal part of the stomach

nized by EUS. EUS appears to be adeqeate for follow-up after surgery and after radio- and/or chemotherapy. Early gastric carcinoma that develops after a combined treatment (irradiation and chemotherapy) for NHL of the stomach can be detected with EUS. Similar observations of metachronous adenocarcinoma after extensive chemo- or radiotherapy have been reported in the literature [20–23]. Fibrotic changes after radio- or chemotherapy cannot always be differentiated sonographically from remaining malignancy. Therefore, the possibility of using EUS-guided biopsy or cytology to make the final diagnosis should further enhance the diagnostic value of this ultrasonic procedure in the future.

References

1. Herrmann R, Panahou AM, Barcos MP, et al. (1980) Gastrointestinal involvement in non-Hodgkins's lymphoma. Cancer 46: 215–222
2. Dawson IMP, Conners YS, Morson BC (1961) Primary malignant lymphoid tumor of the intestinal tract. Br J Surg 49: 80–89
3. Musschoff K (1977) Klinische Studieneinteilung der Nicht-Hodgkin Lymphoma. Strahlentherapie 153: 218–222
4. Van der Werf-Messing BHP (1987) Radiotherapy of extranodal Non-Hodgkin's Lymphoma. Lymphoid Neoplasia II, e. d. Mathe G, Seligman and Tubiana M. Springer Verlag
5. Taal BG, den Hartog Jager FCA, Tytgat GNJ (1987) The endoscopic spectrum of primary non-Hodgkin lymphoma of the stomach. Endoscopy 19: 190–192
6. Spinelli P, Lo Gullo C, Pizzetti P (1980) Endoscopic diagnosis of gastric lymphomas. Endoscopy 12: 211–214   ,
7. Solidoro A, Salazar F, de la Flor J, Sanchez J (1981) Endoscopic tissue diagnosis of gastric involvement in the staging of non-Hodgkin lymphoma. Cancer 48: 1053–1057
8. Kressel HY, Callen PW, Montagne YP, Korobkin M (1978) Computed tomographic evaluation of disorders affecting the alimentary tract. Radiology 129: 451–455
9. Lee KR, Levine E, Moffat RE, et al. (1979) Computed tomographic staging of malignant gastric neoplasms. Radiology 133: 151–155
10. Crone-Münzbrock W, Brockmann WP (1982) Computertomographische und sonographische Diagnostik und Verlaufskontrolle beim malignen Lymphom des Magens. Fortschr Röntgenstr 139: 676–686
11. Lux G, Heyder N, Lutz H, et al. (1982) Endoscopic ultrasonography – technique, orientation and diagnostic possibilities. Endoscopy 14: 220–225
12. Tio TL, Tytgat GNJ (1984) Endoscopic Ultrasonography in the assessment of intra- and transmural infiltration of tumours in the esophagus, stomach and papilla of Vater and in the detection of extraesophageal lesions. Endoscopy 16: 203–210
13. Tio TL, Tytgat GNJ (1986) Endoscopic ultrasonography of normal and pathologic upper gastrointestinal wall structure. Comparison of studies in vivo and in vitro with histology. Scand J Gastroenterol 21: 27–33
14. Tio TL, Tytgat GNJ (1986) Endoscopic ultrasonography in analysing periintestinal lymph node abnormality. Preliminary results of studies in vivo and in vitro. Scand J Gastroenterol (suppl 123) 21: 158–163
15. Tio TL, Tytgat GNJ (1986) Atlas of transintestinal ultrasonography. Mur-Kostverloren. Aalsmeer. The Netherlands
16. Tio TL, den Hartog-Jager FCA, Tytgat GNJ (1986) Endoscopic ultrasonography of Non-Hodgkin Lymphoma of the stomach. Gastroenterology 91: 401–408
17. Aibe T, Ito T, Yoshida T, et al. (1986) Endoscopic ultrasonography of lymph nodes surrounding the upper GI tract. Scand J Gastroenterol (suppl 123): 164–170
18. Aibe T, Fuji T, Okita K, Takemoto T (1986) A fundamental study of normal layer structure of the gastrointestinal wall visualized by endoscopic ultrasonography. Scand J Gastroenterol (suppl 123) 21: 6–15

19. Musschoff K, Schmidt-Vollmer H (1975) Prognosis of Non-Hodgkin's lymphoma with special emphasis in the staging classification. Z Krebsforsch 83: 323–341
20. Ettinger DS, Carter D (1977) Gastric carcinoma 16 years after gastric lymphoma irradiations. Am J Gastroenterol 68: 485–488
21. Shani A, Schutt AJ, Weiland LH (1978) Primary gastric malignant lymphoma followed by gastric adenocarcinoma. Cancer 42: 2039–2044
22. Brumback RA, Gerber JE, Hicks DG, Straucher JA (1984) Adenocarcinoma of the stomach following irradiation and chemotherapy for lymphoma in young patients. Cancer 54: 994–998
23. Beverly WB, Bitter MA, Barm JM, Betwick DG (1987) Gastric Adenocarcinoma after Gastric Lymphoma. Cancer 60: 1876–1882

XII Endoscopic Ultrasonography in the Evaluation of Smooth Muscle Tumors of the Upper Gastrointestinal Tract: A Comparison with Computed Tomography, Endoscopy, and Barium Meal

Introduction

Submucosal gastrointestinal (GI) tumors are usually detected by the double contrast barium meal because of a double contour or by a smooth margined filling defect in the barium column. Distinction between a benign and malignant lesion may be difficult or impossible [1–5]. With endoscopy a submucosal neoplasma is visualized as a bulge covered with normal mucosa or occasionally associated with a central ulcer [6, 7]. Endoscopic biopsy may not be helpful in ascertaining the diagnosis because the lesion cannot always be reached with a standard biopsy forceps without using special techniques [8].

Computed tomography (CT) may identify a submucosal tumor as a hypodense lesion immediately adjacent to the lumen or by thickening of the GI wall after filling the lumen with contrast medium [10–14]. Endoscopic ultrasonography (EUS) is considered to be accurate in detecting and staging of GI neoplasms by directly approaching the target lesion with a high-frequency ultrasonic beam via the GI lumen [15–19].

The aim of this study was to assess the accuracy and limitations of EUS in the detection and staging of smooth muscle tumors in the upper GI tract, by comparing EUS findings to those of CT, barium meal, and histology of resected tissue.

Materials and Methods

Between December 1983 and March 1988 EUS was performed in 26 patients in whom a smooth muscle tumor was suspected after endoscopic or radiographic examination. The patients were divided into three groups. The first group consisted of eight patients who underwent surgery for an extensive lesion which was thought to be benign (group 1). The second group consisted of eight patients who underwent surgery because of suspected malignancy (group 2). The third group consisted of 14 patients with less extensive, sharply delineated lesions, thought to be benign, who did not undergo surgery but were followed-up with EUS and endoscopy (group 3). The results of EUS were correlated with the results of endoscopy and barium meal and also with CT scanning and detailed histological examination of resection specimens when available. A diagnosis of benign lesion was made with EUS when sharply demarcated hypoechoic homogeneous tumors without evidence of penetration into the surrounding tissue or lymph node involvement were recognized. A diagnosis of malignant lesion was made when a bizzarely demarcated, hypoechoic, inhomogeneous mass with evidence of lymph node involvement or a clearly demarcated hypoechoic inhomogeneous tumor without or with penetration into the adjacent gastrointestinal wall but associated with an central ulcerative lesion or a fistula was visualized. Analysis of the accuracy of the EUS interpretation was based either upon histology or upon long-term follow-up.

All studies were performed with a prototype or a commercially available Olympus echoendoscope, which has been described elsewhere [17–21]. The frequency of the transducer is 7.5 MHz and it has a penetration depth of approximately 10 cm and an axial resolution of 0.2 mm. In the last two patients with leiomyosarcomas (group 2) EUS was performed with a prototype Olympus echoendoscope with a frequency of 10 MHz. The penetration depth of the ultrasound is 5 cm with an axial resolution of 0.1 mm. The echoprobe was routinely covered with a water-filled balloon to improve ultrasonic images by making optimal contact with the mucosa. This balloon method was particularly useful for the investigation of the esophagus, the cardia, and the pylorus region. Filling the gastric lumen with water facilitated clear visualization of the gastric wall structures in all other areas. Lesions which could not be adequately coated with water were investigated using both methods. Complications were not encountered in this study.

Results

Table 1 summarizes the results of EUS, CT, endoscopy, barium meal, and histology of the resection specimens (group 1).

Table 1. Summary of the results of EUS, CT, endoscopy, barium meal, and histology of the resection specimens (group 1)

No. of patients	Localization	EUS	CT	Endoscopy	Barium meal	Histology
2	Esophagus	Sharply demarcated homogeneous hypo-echoic lesion or local thickening of the muscularis propria	Hypodense tumor	Bulge with normal mucosa	Filling defect	Leiomyoma
1	Esophagus	Sharply delineated hypoechoic tumor in the submucosa	Hypodense tumor	Bulge with normal mucosa	Filling defect	Carcinoid metastasis
1	Stomach	Sharply demarcated hypoechoic tumor	Aortic aneurysma	No abnor-mality	No abnor-mality	Leiomyoma
2	Stomach	Sharply demarcated hypoechoic tumor with anechoic ductal structures	Hypodense tumor	Bulge with normal mucosa	Filling defect	Leiomyoma with blood vessels
2	Stomach	Local thickening of the muscularis propria	Thickening of the wall	Bulge with normal mucosa	Filling defect	Leiomyoma

In group 1 EUS showed sharply demarcated hypoechoic tumors without ($n = 4$) or with ($n = 2$) some duct-like anechoic structures strongly indicative of blood vessels within the mass. Local thickening of the muscularis propria protruding into the water-filled gastric lumen ($n = 1$) or extending into the perigastric tissue ($n = 1$) was also seen. CT scanning revealed hypodense massess adjacent to the lumen ($n = 6$). In one patient CT did not show a mural abnormality because of the presence of an aortic aneurysm. Endoscopy showed bulges covered with normal mucosa ($n = 6$). Barium meal showed filling defect or double contour. Histology of the resection specimens confirmed the EUS findings in characterizing the size, extent, and the presence of blood vessels. A diagnosis of leiomyoma was made in seven patients. In one patient, however, carcinoid metastasis adjacent to the esophagus was diagnosed.

Table 2 summarizes the results of EUS, CT, endoscopy, barium meal, and histology of the resection specimens or the transmural biopsy (group 2). In group 2 EUS showed a bizarrely demarcated hypoechoic inhomogeneous tumor with some hyperechoic

Table 2. Summary of the results of EUS, CT, endoscopy, barium meal, and histology of the specimens (group 2)

No. of patients	Locali-zation	EUS	CT	Endoscopy	Barium meal	Histology/surgery
1	Esophagus	Bizarrely demarcated inhomogeneous mass with hyperechoic structures (air)	Hypodense mass	Ulcerative tumor with a fistula	Tumor with a deep fistula	Leiomyo-sarcoma with a fistula
1	Esophagus	Hypoechoic mass with suspicious adjacent lymph nodes	Hypodense mass adjacent to the lumen	Bulge covered with normal mucosa	Filling defect	Bronchus carcinoma
2	Stomach	Bizarrely delineated mass adjacent to the liver or spleen	Hypodense mass directly adjacent to the liver or spleen	Bulge covered with normal mucosa	Double contrast	Non-resect-able leiomyo-sarcoma
2	Stomach	Clearly demarcated hypoechoic mass with a central ulcerative lesion	Not per-formed	Bulge with an ulcer	Double con-tour mass a central ulcer	Leiomyo-blastoma, leomyo-sarcoma
2	Stomach	Clearly demarcated hypoechoic mass with suspicious lymph nodes	Hypodense mass	Bulge with a central ulcer	Double contour with a central ulcer	Leiomyo-sarcoma with (1) and without (1) adjacent lymph node metastasis

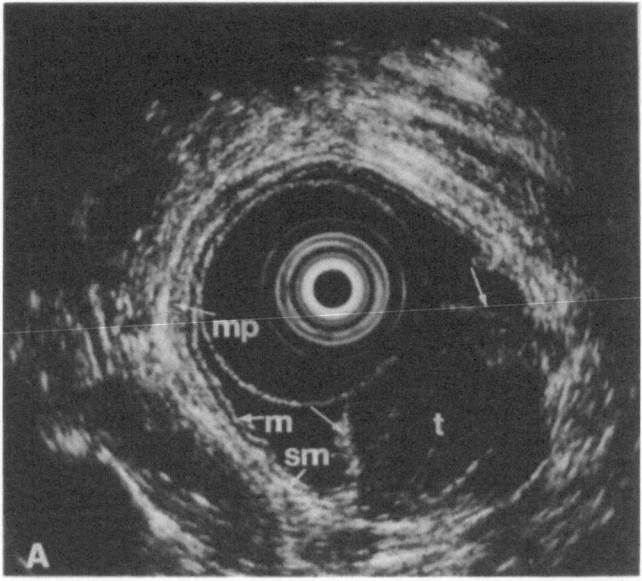

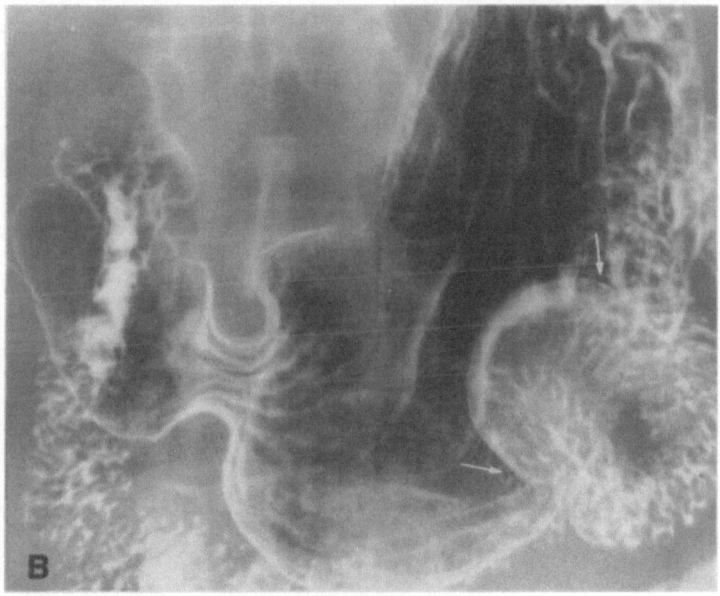

Fig. 1. A EUS image shows a polypoid well delineated hypochoic homogeneous tumor mass *(t)* without penetration into the surrounding tissues protruding into the gastric lumen (arrows) m = mucosa, sm = submucosa, mp = muscularis propria. **C** CT-scan image shows a hypodense, clearly delineated tumor mass *(t)* adjacent to the gastric lumen *(lu)*. **B** Barium meal image shows five smooth marginated filling defects with sharply demarcated margins

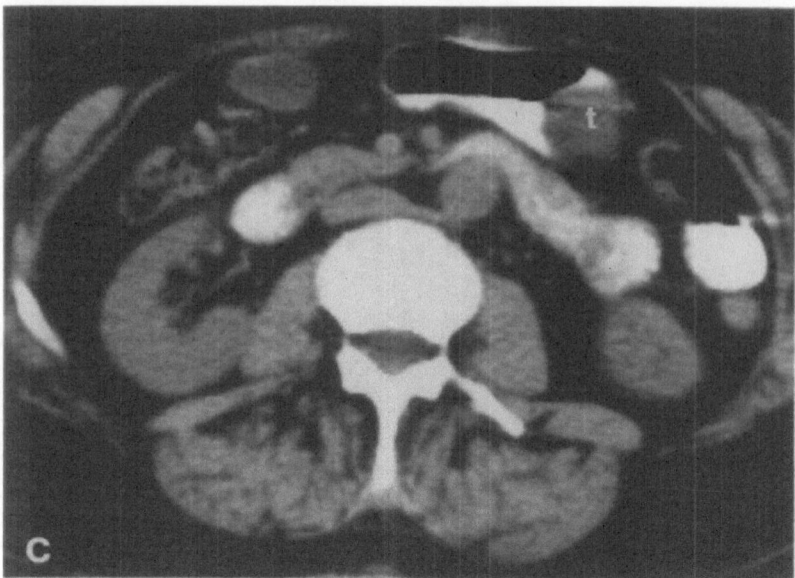

Fig. 1

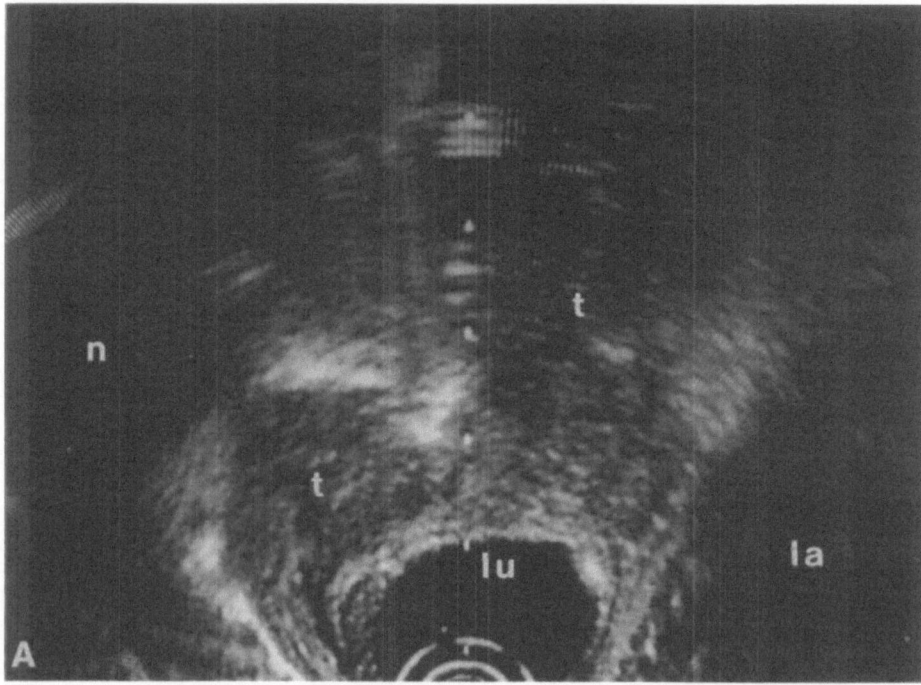

Fig. 2. A EUS image shows a semicircular hypoechoic lesion *(t)* with deep penetration into the surrounding tissues and presence of a hyperechoic structure within the tumor mass carrows compatible with air accumulation due to a fistula. **B** Barium swallow shows a marrowing of the esophageal lumen (arrow) with a deep fistula *(f)*. **C** Histology of the resection specimen shows a large tissue mass *(t)* penetrating through the muscularis propria with destruction Carrows of the overlying mucosa *(m)*.

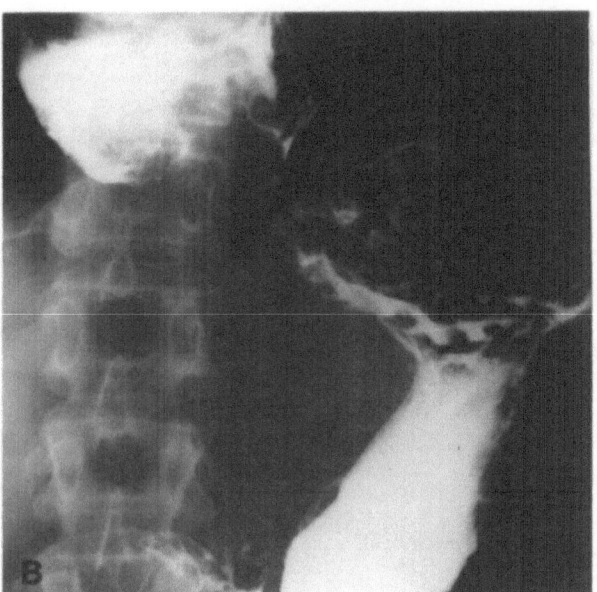

Fig. 2

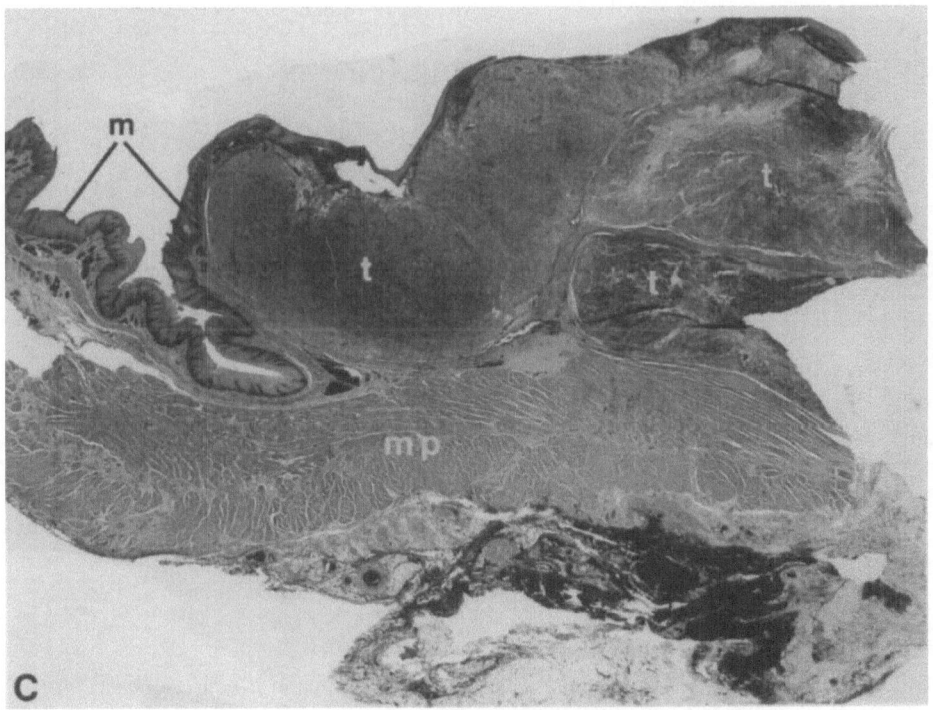

Fig. 2

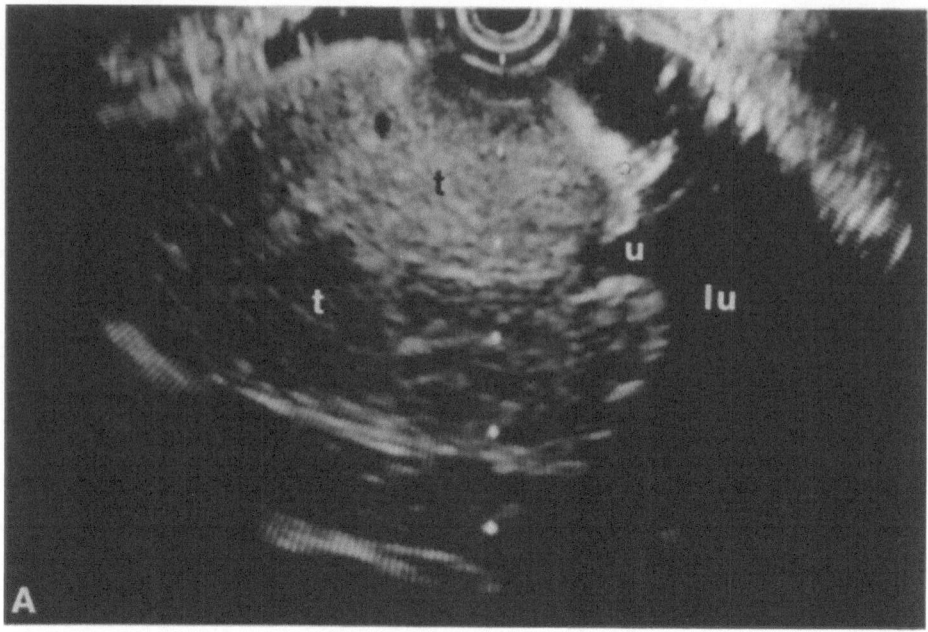

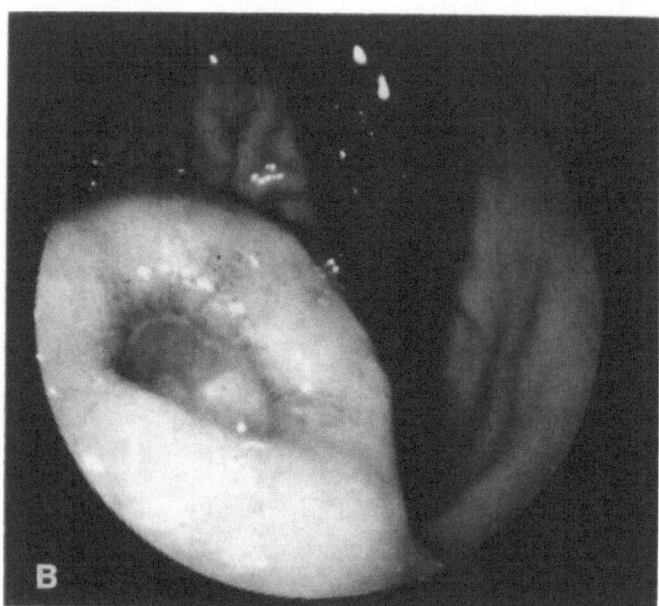

Fig. 3. A EUS image shows a longituchinal section of an extensive tumor *(t)* with central ulcer *(u)*. lu = lumen, **B** Corresponding endosurgy shows the tumor mass *(t)* with an ulcerative defect *(u)*. **C** Corresponding histology of the resection specimen reveals a leiomyosarcoma *(t)* with ulceration *(u)*.

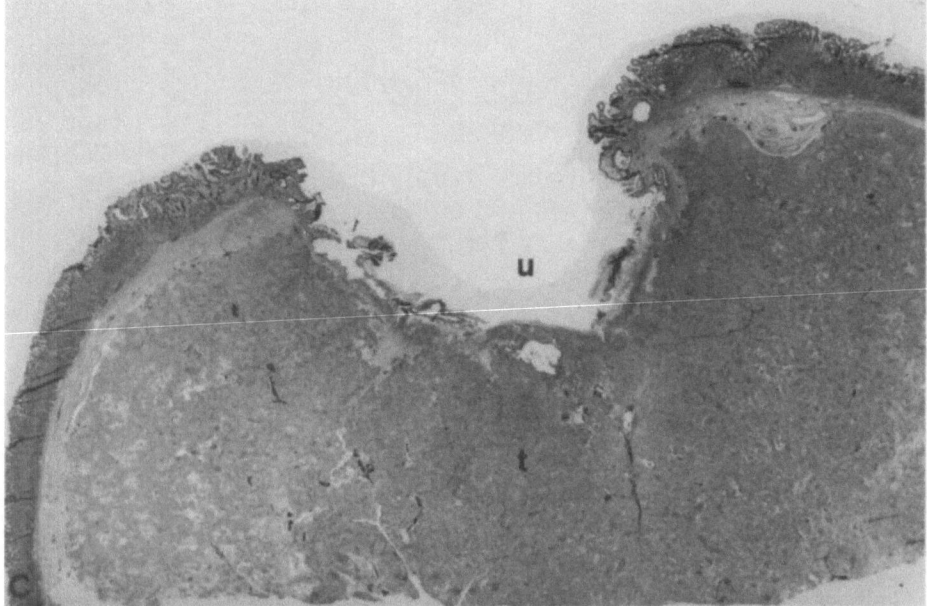

Fig. 3

structures strongly indicative of the presence of air within the mass in the esophagus ($n = 1$). Deeply penetrated hypoechoic masses with suspicious adjacent lymph nodes bordering the bronchus ($n = 1$) or the liver ($n = 1$) or the spleen ($n = 1$) were also detected. CT revealed hypodense masses adjacent to the GI lumen ($n = 4$). Endoscopy and barium meal showed an esophageal tumor with a fistula -($n = 1$) or bulges covered with smooth mucosa ($n = 3$). Histology of the resection specimen of the first patient enabled the diagnosis of leiomyosarcoma in the esophagus with a fistula. In the last three patients the tumor was proven to be nonresectable at surgery because of deep penetration into the adjacent structures. Histology of the transmural biopsy resulted in diagnoses of bronchus carcinoma ($n = 1$) and leiomyosarcoma ($n = 2$). EUS showed sharply demarcated inhomogeneous tumors with central ulcerative lesions ($n = 4$). Adjacent lymph nodes strongly suspicious of metastasis were found ($n = 2$). CT showed hypodense tumors ($n = 2$). Endoscopy and barium meal showed bulges or double contours with antral ulcers ($n = 4$). Histology of the resection specimens enabled diagnoses of leiomyoblastoma ($n = 1$) and leiomyosarcoma ($n = 3$) to be made. Lymph node metastasis was found in one of these patients.

During follow-up after surgical resection (range 12–24 months $n = 5$) only EUS revealed mural and nodal abnormalities ($n = 3$). EUS demonstrated a deeply penetrated hypoechoic mass adjacent to the liver with adjacent lymph node involvement ($n = 1$). CT failed to register the intramural abnormality. Histology of the transcutaneous guided puncture showed leiomyosarcoma. EUS revealed a circumscribed hypoechoic lesion adjacent to the site of previous fundectomy ($n = 1$). CT showed thickening of the gastric wall. Histology of the resection specimen resulted in the

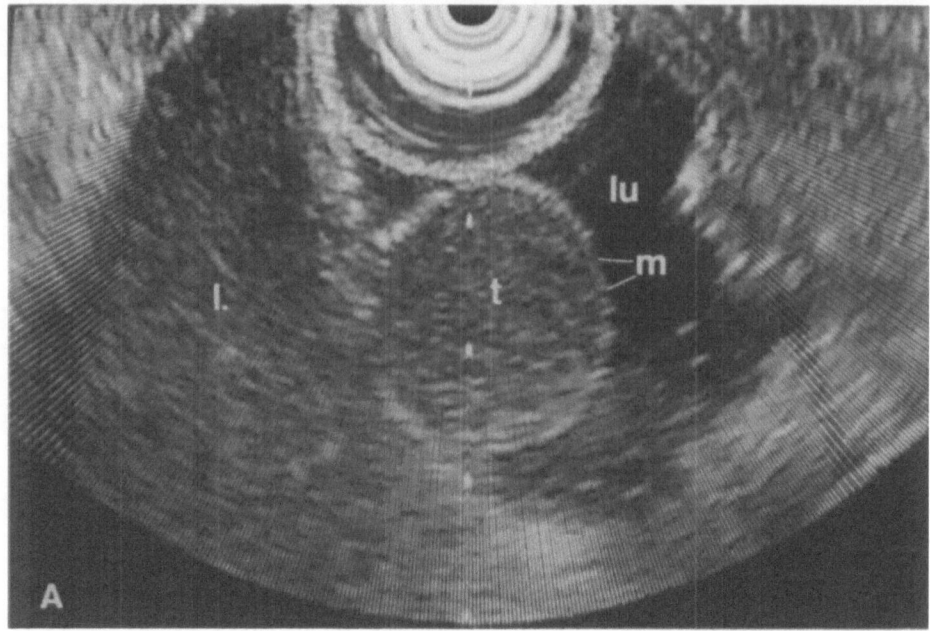

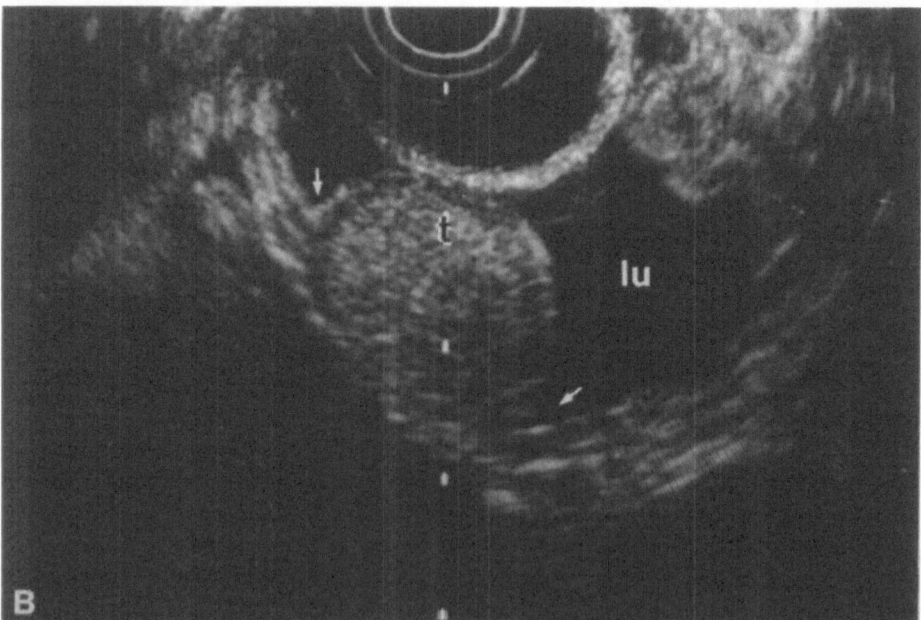

Fig. 4. A Initial EUS image shows a sharply delineated hypoechoic lesion *(t)* protruding into the gastric lumen *(lu)* directly adjacent to the liver *(l)*. **B** Follow-up EUS picture shows no changes of size, boundaries and echo pattern of the tumor *(t)* protruding into the gastric lumen. *(lu)*. l = liver. **C** Corresponding barium swallow shows bulging of the wall covered with normal mucosa.

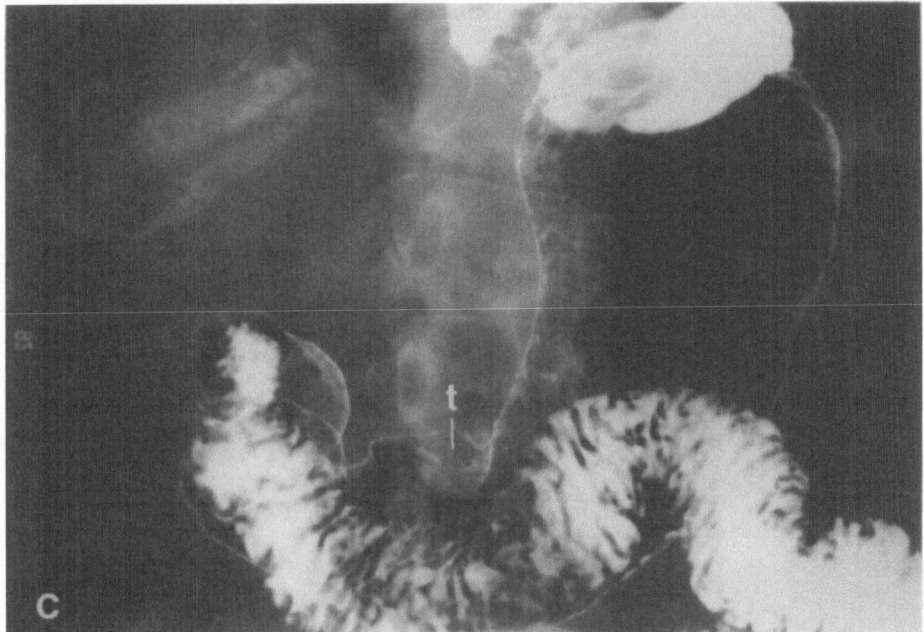

Fig. 4

diagnosis of leiomyosarcoma in the omentum without evidence of malignancy in the gastric wall. In the last three patients EUS did not show evidence of recurrence.

Table 3 summarizes the results of endoscopy, barium meal, CT scanning, and initial and follow-up EUS (group 3).

In group 3 endoscopy revealed bulges covered with normal mucosa in the esophagus ($n = 4$), stomach ($n = 8$), and duodenum ($n = 2$). Barium meal showed a filling defect or double contour. CT demonstrated wall thickening. Initial EUS showed sharply demarcated hypoechoic lesions ($n = 6$) or local thickening of the muscularis propria ($n = 8$) beyond the normal overlying mucosa and submucosa. During follow-up (range 1–3 years) EUS did not reveal changes in size, extent, and echopattern of the tumor.

Discussion

EUS is accurate in the detection and staging of smooth muscle tumors in the GI tract because it enables the intestinal wall structure to be analyzed in detail. Criteria allowing identification of a leiomyoma are local thickening of the muscularis propria or the presence of a mass lesion with a homogeneous, sharply delineated echopattern covered with normal mucosa and submucosa. Occasionally a central ulcer may be found within the mass. A leiomyosarcoma or a leiomyoblastoma is visualized as an inhomogeneous hypoechoic tumor mass usually with bizzarely shaped but clearly demarcated boundaries and often associated with an ulcerous defect or fistulous tract.

Table 3. Summary of the results of endoscopy, barium meal, CT, initial EUS and follow-up (FU) (group 3)

No. of patients	Localization	Endoscopy	Barium meal	CT	EUS (initial)	FU
4	Esophagus	Bulge with normal mucosa	Filling defect	Local thickening of the wall (2) no abnormalities (2)	Sharply demarcated hypoechoic pattern (2), local thickening of the muscularis propria (2)	No changes in size and echopattern
8	Stomach	Bulge with normal mucosa	Double contour	No abnormality in 1 out of 3 patients	Sharply demarcated hypoechoic pattern (6), local thickening of the muscularis propria (2)	No changes in size and echopattern
2	Duodenum	Bulge with normal mucosa	Filling defect (1), no abnormality (1)	No abnormality	Local thickening of the muscularis propria (2)	No changes in size and echopattern

Supplementary findings such as penetration into the surrounding tissue or the presence of suspicious lymph nodes are helphul in recognizing the malignant nature of the lesion.

EUS appears to be superior to other methods not only in detection and staging of smooth muscle tumors but also during follow-up after resection of malignant tissue. Endoscopy and barium meal can only show mucosal abnormalities. Even CT scanning is frequently inadequate for detecting intramural lesion because of the lack of resolution in precisely defining the intestinal wall structure. Moreover, blood vessels within or adjacent to the mass can be difficult to distinguish from the primary lesion with CT because of the static character of the procedure [22]. In contrast, the real-time dynamic properties of EUS enable accurate differentiation between solid lesions such as tumor masses and lymph nodes and blood vessels; in addition, cross and longitudinal section of lesions can be obtained by endoscopic maneuvering of the echoprobe. This ist of utmost importance because CT can make only cross sections. Lymph nodes immediately adjacent to the gastric wall can be clearly visualized by EUS. Difficulties may be encountered in differentiating leiomyoma from metastatic lesions in the submucosa, e. g. carcinoid metastasis or bronchogenic carcinoma penetrating into the adjacent esophageal wall, from leiomyosarcoma because of the similar appearance of the echopattern of each disease. Therefore, the final diagnosis can only be made by histology. The possibility of using the biopsy channel for EUS-guided biopsy or cytological puncture may further enhance the diagnostic value of this new diagnostic modality.

EUS also has some disadvantages over conventional imaging modalities. It may be difficult for the operator to interpret the ultrasonic images because of the difficulty in adequately positioning the echoprobe on the target lesions. The operator must have extensive experience of both endoscopy and ultrasonography. CT scanning is superior to EUS in detecting lymph nodes distant to the GI lumen because of the limited penetration depth of the ultrasonic beam [16].

In the near future EUS may become an important diagnostic procedure in gastroenterology. When abnormalities of the GI wall are found endoscopically, the EUS probe can be placed on the lesion to evaluate the mural extent and the probable origin of the neoplasm. The presence or absence of perigastrointestinal lymph node involvement can also be determined. EUS may even show the optimal site from which biopsy or cytology specimens can be obtained.

References

1. Baker HL, Good CA (1955) Smooth muscle tumors of the alimentary tract. Their roentgen manifestations. Amer J Roentgen 74: 246–254
2. Phillips JC, Lindsay JW, Kendall JA (1970) Gastric leiomyosarcoma: roentgenologic and clinical findings. Amer J Dig Dis 15: 239–246
3. Fargenburg D, Farman J, Dallemand S, et al. (1975) Leiomyoblastoma of the stomach. Report of 9 cases. Radiology 117: 297–300
4. Welch JP (1975) Smooth muscle tumors of the stomach. Amer J Surg 130: 279–285
5. Nauert TC, Zornoza J, Ordonez N (1982) Gastric leiomyosarcomas. Am J R 139: 291–297
6. Faivre J, Bory R, Moulinier B (1978) Benign tumors of oesophagus: value of endoscopy. Endoscopy 10: 264–268
7. Papazian A, Gineston JL, Capron JP, Quenum C (1984) Leiomyoblastoma of the stomach: endoscopic treatment. Endoscopy 16: 157–159
8. Kaneko E, Kumagai J, Honda N, et al. (1983) Evaluation of the new giantbiopsy forceps in the diagnosis of mucosal and submucosal gastric lesions. Endoscopy 15: 322-326
9. Balfe DM, Koehler RE, Karstaedt N, et al. (1981) Computed tomography of gastric neoplasms. Radiology 140: 431–436
10. Pillazi G, Weinzeb J, Vernace F, et al. (1983) CT of gastric masses: image pattern and a note on potential pitfalls. Gastrointest Radiol 8: 11–17
11. McLeod AJ, Zornoza J, Shirkoda A (1984) Leiomyosarcoma: computed tomography findings. Radiology 152: 133–136
12. Scatarige JC, Fishman EK, Jones B, et al. (1985) Gastric leiomyosarcoma: CT observations. J Comput Assist Tomorg 9: 320–327
13. Megibow AJ, Balthazar EJ, Hulnick DH, et al. (1985) CT evaluation of gastrointestinal leiomyomas and leiomyosarcomas AJR 144: 727–731
14. Tio TL, Tytgat GNJ (1984) Endoscopic ultrasonography in the assessment of intra- and transmural infiltration of tumours in the oesophagus, stomach and papilla of Vater and in the detection of extraoesophageal lesions. Endoscopy 16: 203–210
15. Tio TL, Tytgat GNJ (1986) Endoscopic ultrasonography of normal and pathologic upper gastrointestinal wall structure. Comparison of studies in vivo and in vitro with histology. Scand J Gastroenterol 21 (suppl 123): 27–33
16. Tio TL, den Hartog Jager FCA, Tytgat GNJ (1986) Endoscopic ultrasonography of Non-Hodgkin lymphoma of the stomach. Gastroenterology 91: 401–408
17. Tio TL, den Hartog Jager FCA, Tytgat GNJ (1986) The role of endoscopic ultrasonography in assessing local resectability of oesophagogastric malignancies. Accuracy, pitfalls, an predictability. Scand J Gastroenterol 21 (suppl 123): 78–86

18. Tio TL, Tytgat GNJ (1986) Atlas of Transintestinal Ultrasonography. Mur-Kostverloren, Aals-meer, The Netherlands
19. Yasuda K, Nakajima M, Kawai K (1986) Endoscopic ultrasonography in the diagnosis of submucosal tumor of the upper digestive tract. Scand J Gastroenterol 21 (suppl 123): 59–67
20. Di Magno EP, Regan PT, Clain JE, et al. (1982) Human endoscopic ultrasonography. Gastroen-terology 83: 824–829
21. Lux G, Heyder N, Lutz H, et al. (1982) Endoscopic ultrasonography-technique, orientation and diagnostic possibilities. Endoscopy 14: 220–225
22. Herlinger H (1966) The recognition of exogastric tumours. Report of six cases. Br J Radiol 39: 25–36
23. Evans HL (1985) Smooth muscle tumors of the gastrointestinal wall. A study of 56 cases followed for a minimum of 10 years. Cancer 56: 2242–2250

Summary

Endoscopic ultrasonography (EUS) is a fascinating combination of two high technologies – endoscopy and ultrasound – in which a small echoprobe is attached to the tip of a side-viewing endoscope. By directly approaching the target lesion with a high-frequency real-time ultrasonic beam via the intestinal lumen, a new dimension of ultrasonic resolution can be obtained.

In the *first* chapter the investigative technique is described. The technique of EUS investigation of the upper GI tract is similar to that of any other endoscopic method, and it involves intravenous sedation and pharyngeal anesthesia. The target lesion should be reached endoscopically and then visualized sonographically by filling the balloon attached to the tip of the instrument with water or by filling the GI lumen with water. Cross, longitudinal, and oblique sections should be made for accurate assessment of the lesion. In the esophagus, only the water-filled balloon method can be used. In the stomach, the water-filled stomach method is best for clear visualization of the intraluminal extent of lesions. Because of the anatomic tomographic relationship between the pancreas and the stomach, the splenic vein should be used as an orientation landmark for accurate visualization of the entire organ. The portal vein should be used as a landmark for visualization of the biliary tree. For evaluation of rectosigmoid lesions, the prostate or the uterus, the bladder, and the coccygeal bone can be used as orientating landmarks. For assessing rectal and perirectal diseases, a rigid or flexible nonendoscopic ultrasonic instrument can be used. For rectosigmoid lesions, however, an endoscopic ultrasonic instrument is preferable.

In the *second* chapter an in vitro study of EUS (autopsy and resection specimen) in interpreting the GI wall is described. The wall is seen as a five-layer structure. Although the interpretation of the mucosa is still debatable and needs further evaluation, the interpretation of the submucosa and muscularis propria is generally accepted and allows differentiation between early and advanced carcinoma of the upper GI tract.

In the *third* chapter the interpretation of periintestinal lymph node abnormalities is described. Lymph nodes are visualized as round or ellipsoid structures adjacent to the intestinal wall. Lymph nodes with a hypoechoic echopattern similar to or more hypoechoic than the primary lesion with sharply demarcated boundaries are strongly indicative of malignancy. In contrast, lymph nodes with a more hypoechoic pattern than the primary lesion and nonsharply delineated boundaries are strongly indicative of inflammatory changes. Micrometastases or granulomatous inflammation are often difficult to distinguish from malignant lesions.

In the *fourth* chapter the preoperative staging of esophagogastric malignancy with EUS in comparison with histology is described. Curative resectability is shown by a hypoechoic intramural lesion without penetration into the muscularis propria with or without regional lymph node involvement. Palliative resection is described by hypoechoic intramural echopattern without deep penetration into the surrounding tissue usually associated with adjacent lymph node involvement. Non resectability is shown by hypoechoic mural infiltration with deep penetration into the surrounding tissues, e. g., major blood vessels. Overall, a high degree of accuracy is obtained in assessing the depth of tumor infiltration and the presence of lymph node involvement. Differentiation between early and advanced cancer is possible. Stenosis, however, is a definitive limiting factor. Differentiation between benign and malignant lymph nodes can occasionally be difficult. Using the biopsy channel for ultrasound-guided puncture and reducing the length of the rigid tip may further enhance the accuracy of EUS.

In the *fifth* chapter preoperative staging of pancreatic and periampullary malignant tumors is described. EUS enables accurate determination of the extent of the lesions and the presence of suspicious lymph node involvement. Curative resection is indicated by the presence of clearly demarcated hypoechoic tumor without evidence of lymph node involvement. The presence of suspicious lymph nodes is indicative of palliative resectability. Carcinomas deeply invading the surrounding major blood vessels suggest nonresectability.

In the *sixth* chapter preoperative staging of malignant bile duct tumors is described. The usual EUS findings consisted of intraductal mass lesions with adjacent lymph node involvement. It is necessary to know the depth of tumor infiltration into the surrounding tissue to assess local resectability. A clearly demarcated hypoechoic malignant growth with or without evidence of regional lymph node involvement is indicative of local curative resectability. Involvement of distant lymph nodes is thought to be indicative of palliative resectability. Evidence of deep penetration into the surrounding tissues, e. g., major blood vessels or organs, is considered to be indicative of nonresectability.

In the *seventh* chapter an arterious malformation in a gastric polyp is described. The vascular abnormality was clearly visualized as an anechoic structure prior to endoscopic removal of the polyp. Although endoscopic coagulation of the pedicle proceeded slowly and with the utmost care causing apparently adequate coagulation of the stalk, the depth of coagulation appeared to be insufficient to prevent major hemorrhage. From this experience, EUS examination of the pedicle of large polyps to identify the size of the vessels is recommended.

In the *eighth* chapter EUS of non-Hodgkin lymphoma of the stomach in eight patients is described. Findings consisted of intramural infiltration or mucosal alteration with perigastric lymph nodes involvement, or both. EUS was more accurate than computed tomography (CT) in the detection of the transmural extent of malignancy and adjacent lymph node involvement. Because of the limited penetration depth of ultrasound, more distant lymph nodes, however, can be more clearly visualized with CT. Infiltration beyond the normal underlying mucosa may readily be recognized with EUS. This is of utmost importance, particularly for those patients who do not have endoscopic or radiographic evidence of mucosal involvement. EUS appears to be superior not only in detection but also in follow-up, as endoscopy and barium meal studies can only show mucosal abnormalities. Technical improvements such as EUS-guided cytological puncture or biopsy are recommended.

In the *ninth* chapter a comparison is made of blind transrectal ultrasonography (BUS) and endoscopic transrectal ultrasonography in assessing rectal and perirectal diseases. BUS and EUS are both adequate in staging advanced rectal cancer. EUS is more accurate than BUS in assessing small tumors localized in the mucosa and submucosa. Adjacent lymph node abnormality is more clearly visualized with EUS because of the high resolution of this instrument, using a 7.5-MHz ultrasonic beam. In contrast, distant lymph node involvement is more clearly visualized with BUS because of the penetration depth of the 5-MHz ultrasonic beam. Differentiation between villous adenoma and villous adenoma with malignancy can more accurately be made with EUS. Perirectal disease can be more clearly visualized with BUS. Further studies in a large number of patients are recommended.

In the *tenth* chapter evaluation of resectability of gastrointestinal tumors is described. In this review article benign and malignant tumors of the esophagus, stomach, and the biliopancreatic system are discussed. In the preoperative assessment of resectability criteria are used which were described in the previous chapter. Data collected in tables support the value of EUS preoperative staging of malignant GI tumors. Moreover, smooth muscle tumors of the esophagus and stomach are described. In the preoperative staging of esophagogastric malignant tumors EUS appears to be superior to CT because the depth of infiltration, the longitudinal extent, and the presence of lymph node abnormalities can be visualized. Moreover, the real-time properties of EUS allow clear visualization of vascular involvement and distinguishing of blood vessels from lymph nodes. Stenosis which cannot be passed by the echoendoscope is considered to be a definitive limiting factor. EUS is also accurate in staging biliopancreatic tumors because it enable visualization of both ductal and parenchymal abnormalities together with adjacent lymph node involvement. Difficulties may arise in distinguishing inflammation from malignant infiltration.

In the *eleventh* chapter evaluation of non-Hodgkin lymphoma with EUS, CT, endoscopy, and barium meal in 31 patients according the modified Ann-Arbor system and the endoscopic pattern are described. Stage I and stage II disease are correctly diagnosed only with EUS. Stage III disease is correctly diagnosed with both techniques. Stage IV disease, however, is diagnosed more accurately with CT than with EUS because of the limited penetration depth of ultrasound. An early gastric carcinoma was found after successful treatment. Twenty-two patients treated with chemotherapy were evaluated with EUS and endoscopy before and after treatment. The correlations between the three endoscopic patterns and EUS findings are described.

In the *twelfth* chapter EUS is compared with CT, endoscopy, and barium meal in the evaluation of smooth muscle tumors of the upper GI tract. Ten patients suspected of having leiomyoma and ten patients suspected of having leiomyomasarcoma were studied by EUS, CT, endoscopy, and barium meal prior to surgery. The results were correlated with histology: 9 leiomyomas, 1 carcinoid metastatis, 6 leiomyosarcomas, 1 leiomyoblastoma, 1 mesothelioma, 1 mucous secreting adenocarcinoma, and 1 bronchus carcinoma were diagnosed by histology. Nineteen patients suspected of having leiomyoma from the results of endoscopy, barium meal, or CT were available for study. A leiomyoma is diagnosed with EUS by the presence of thickening of the muscularis propria or a clearly demarcated hypoechoic homogeneous tumor. A leiomyoblastoma is diagnosed by the presence of a extensive hypoechoic inhomogeneous mass with irregular boundaries or lack of margination or a clearly delineated hypoechoic mass with central ulcer or a fistula. Occasionally, suspicious lymph nodes adjacent to the mass can be found. EUS appeared superior to other imaging techniques.

Moreover, follow-up after treatment (chemotherapy, radiotherapy, laser photo-coagulation therapy, surgery) can more accurately be performed than with presently available diagnostic modalities. It has now become reality that selection of patients who should benefit from surgery can be made preoperatively. I hope that explorative laparotomy becomes obsolete and that the cost explosion of medical treatment can be reduced. I belief that EUS will become an important diagnostic tool in gastroenterology. In the near future, the possibility of using the biopsy channel for ultrasound-guided puncture will not only enhance the diagnostic accuracy but also allow one to perform therapeutic procedures such as transintestinal drainage of pancreatic pseudo-cysts or perirectal abscesses. Although the learning period is relative long with this technique, technical improvements and standardization of investigative techniques will make this technique more popular and useful.

In conclusion, I consider that EUS has opened a new diagnostic field to ultrasound, particularly in esophagogastric, rectosigmoid, and periampullary disease. The ability of EUS to show the GI wall structure is such detail and the adequate correlation with histological architecture allows accurate staging of GI tumors according to the TNM classification.